MW01026240

This Should Not Be Happening

YOUNG ADULTS WITH CANCER

by
Anne Katz, PhD, RN

Hygeia Media
An imprint of the Oncology Nursing Society
Pittsburgh, Pennsylvania

ONS Publications Department
Executive Director, Professional Practice and Programs:
Elizabeth M. Wertz Evans, PhD, RN, MPM, CPHQ, CPHIMS, FHIMSS, FACMPE
Director of Publications: Bill Tony, BA, CQIA
Managing Editor: Lisa M. George, BA
Technical Content Editor: Angela D. Klimaszewski, RN, MSN
Staff Editor II: Amy Nicoletti, BA
Copy Editor: Laura Pinchot, BA
Graphic Designer: Dany Sjoen
Editorial Assistant: Judith Holmes

Library of Congress Cataloging-in-Publication Data
Katz, Anne (Anne Jennifer), 1958-
This should not be happening : young adults with cancer / by Anne Katz, PhD, RN.
  pages cm
Includes bibliographical references.
ISBN 978-1-935864-44-8 (alk. paper)
1. Cancer–Popular works. 2. Young adults–Diseases. I. Title.
RC263.K2775 2014
616.99'400835–dc23

2013036935

Publisher's Note

This book is published by the Oncology Nursing Society (ONS). ONS neither represents nor guarantees that the practices described herein will, if followed, ensure safe and effective patient care. The recommendations contained in this book reflect ONS's judgment regarding the state of general knowledge and practice in the field as of the date of publication. The recommendations may not be appropriate for use in all circumstances. Those who use this book should make their own determinations regarding specific safe and appropriate patient-care practices, taking into account the personnel, equipment, and practices available at the hospital or other facility at which they are located. The author and publisher cannot be held responsible for any liability incurred as a consequence from the use or application of any of the contents of this book. Figures and tables are used as examples only. They are not meant to be all-inclusive, nor do they represent endorsement of any particular institution by ONS. Mention of specific products and opinions related to those products do not indicate or imply endorsement by ONS. Websites mentioned are provided for information only; the hosts are responsible for their own content and availability. Unless otherwise indicated, dollar amounts reflect U.S. dollars.

ONS publications are originally published in English. Publishers wishing to translate ONS publications must contact ONS about licensing arrangements. ONS publications cannot be translated without obtaining written permission from ONS. (Individual tables and figures that are reprinted or adapted require additional permission from the original source.) Because translations from English may not always be accurate or precise, ONS disclaims any responsibility for inaccuracies in words or meaning that may occur as a result of the translation. Readers relying on precise information should check the original English version.

Printed in the United States of America

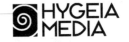

An imprint of the Oncology Nursing Society

For my husband Alan:

With thanks
for the
young adults we once were
and the
ones we have raised

Contents

Foreword

When I was first diagnosed with ovarian cancer in 2003, a month before my 23rd birthday, I had no idea where to turn for information and support. I didn't know anyone else my age with cancer, and the support groups I joined were filled with men and women 30, 40, and 50 years my senior. Always a researcher at heart, I turned to books to help guide me on my journey, but none of the books were written for me. I wanted information on fertility and creating a family after cancer, sex and cancer for young single females, and how to advocate for myself at a time when I hadn't yet learned how to navigate serious illness and didn't have a partner or family close by to help me make sense of treatment options or find resources to support me through my cancer diagnosis.

I mostly muddled through that year on my own, eventually meeting a couple of other young patients with cancer and survivors to whom I could relate. And as the years passed by, cancer became a faded memory, something that had happened but which didn't need to be dealt with as a constant threat on a daily basis. In 2010, that changed, and I was diagnosed with an ovarian cancer recurrence shortly after my 30th birthday.

I thought this time things would have changed and that there would be far more information available to me as a young adult going through a cancer diagnosis for the second time. But in seven years, very little had changed in the landscape of written resources for young adults with cancer. Sure, groups like Stupid Cancer and Young Adult Cancer Canada had been started to support young adults with cancer, but it takes time to find those organizations—I needed a book to tell me they even existed! The Internet is a great place for resources, but it's also scary for a newly diagnosed patient. Many of us avoid reading about our disease, afraid we'll read about statistics and stories that will discourage us. And it can be difficult to know how to tell good information from bad.

I was (and still am) a much better patient the second time around. I know how to advocate for myself and how to navigate patient services. I know that I can access psychosocial and palliative care (and that palliative care doesn't mean I'm dying) and how to look for second opinions and clinical trials. But I had to learn that all on my own. It took being a cancer patient on and off for 10 years to learn *how* to be a cancer patient and how to live beyond a cancer diagnosis.

It has been my sincere hope since that first diagnosis more than a decade ago that young adults faced with a cancer diagnosis would be able to access a book that not only shares stories of others in similar situations but also provides direction on how to access support and how to talk to your doctor, your partner, your family, and your friends; that discusses the physical and emotional changes of a body going through the trauma of illness and treatment; and that faces head-on the reality of recurrence and advanced disease. When I met Dr. Anne Katz at a Young Adult Cancer Canada conference in November 2012, I knew I had met the person to write this book. She understood that facing cancer in your 20s and 30s, when you are just learning how to be an adult, when your career or schooling and relationships are new, or when you're starting a family or dating for the first time, is a very different journey than the one faced by those in their 50s and 60s who have had time to build careers and families and networks of support. So Anne and I sat down and discussed the topics most important to young adults at the beginning of and throughout a cancer diagnosis. From there, the book was born.

It's possible that this book is the first thing you are reading about cancer and dealing with a diagnosis as a young adult. I hope it provides you with guidance and helps direct you to the information and resources you need to be an active participant in your care. I hope it provides you with questions to ask your healthcare team and answers about where to look for support. I hope that the stories shared within make you feel less isolated and show you that you are not alone. Cancer is scary, especially when you are young, but there are things you can do to take control and live beyond your diagnosis. Let this book help guide you, and best of luck on your journey.

Alicia Merchant
10-year ovarian cancer survivor

CHAPTER 1

Introduction

I n North America, more than 70,000 people between the ages of 15 and 39 hear the words "You have cancer" each year (Abramson Cancer Center of the University of Pennsylvania, 2012). Five-year survival rates now reach more than 80%, a significant improvement over the past 20 years (Bleyer, O'Leary, Barr, & Ries, 2006; Canadian Cancer Society Steering Committee, 2009), and more than one million people living now were diagnosed with cancer as young adults. That's a lot of people and a lot of living. It is widely recognized within the oncology community that this group of survivors has needs that differ from those on either side of this age group (children and older adults). But what are those needs, and how are they being met? This book is a response to the question, What do young adults with cancer need to live full lives?

This book is divided into three parts:
I. Being Sick
II. Being a Person
III. Being an Adult.

These divisions are not exact, and overlap exists among chapters and sections. Just like you cannot separate your brain from your heart and the rest of your body, you cannot separate your life with cancer into discrete experiences. But every book needs some organization, and this is what I have tried to do with this book.

In the first section, **Being Sick**, you will read about treatment decision making, the emotional effects of living with cancer, survivorship care and surveillance, fertility and contraception, and living with metastatic disease and preparing for end-of-life care.

In section two, **Being a Person**, you will read about dating and sexuality; exercise, nutrition, and complementary therapies; and psychosocial support and dealing with family and friends.

The final section, **Being an Adult**, contains chapters on issues where you have to stand up and be counted: returning to work or school and participating in research and clinical trials.

Each chapter is based on the latest available evidence from a detailed review of the existing medical, nursing, and psychosocial literature. The goal is to provide you, the reader, with the best information to help you along your journey, either as a patient/survivor or as a family member, friend, spouse, lover, or healthcare provider.

In the appendix you will read the stories, much abbreviated, of the people who were interviewed for this book. There were 18 in total: 16 young adults and 2 mothers of young adults with cancer. You will read their words and learn about their experiences and feelings in textboxes interspersed throughout the book. While the statistics and studies tell part of the story, the words of those who have "been there, done that" are an integral part of what this book aims to do: to describe our essential understanding of cancer in young adults at this time and in this place.

What Is It Like to Have Cancer as a Young Adult?

Many studies have explored this question, and a group of researchers combined the results of 17 studies from 1987–2011 into one comprehensive model (Taylor, Pearce, Gibson, Fern, & Whelan, 2013). From their review, they described nine themes with supporting subthemes, which are presented in Table 1. Albeit coincidentally, the material in this book aligns with these themes and subthemes.

Needs—Met and Unmet

Another way of describing the experience of people with cancer is to explore their needs and to measure which were met, wholly or in part, and which were left unmet (which is not good). Researchers from Australia (Millar, Patterson, & Desille, 2010) did just that: they asked 63 young adults with cancer to respond to a list of 132 needs identified in previous studies. These young adults were asked to identify the 10 most unmet needs based on time since treatment (at or within one year; one to five years; and more than five years). Details of their unmet needs are presented in Tables 2, 3, and 4. What is shocking is the percentage of those who had multiple unmet needs in all three time periods. There is obviously much room for improvement in various aspects of care.

This is a long and frustrating list for those of us who work with young adults because we try our best to meet the needs of those we care for. However, to be living with unmet needs is another matter entirely. It is our fervent hope that this book will help to address, at least in part, many of these unmet needs. So read on—one chapter at a time, one section at a time, as much or as little as you'd like. Feel free to email me (drannekatz@gmail.com) with your thoughts and experiences. Let me know if this book helped, even just a little, and how it could be better.

Table 1. Issues for Young Adults With Cancer	
Theme	**Subthemes**
Psychological function	Changes in appearance Coping General emotional impact
Importance of peers	Communication Friends without cancer Friends with cancer Death of a peer
Experience of health care	Place of care Relationship to professionals Provision of information
Importance of support	Family support Support from friends Support from health professionals General issues related to support
Impact of symptoms	Fatigue Symptoms in general Long-term impact
Striving for normality	—
Impact of diagnosis	—
Positive experiences	—
Financial consequences	Impact on employment State benefits

Note. Based on information from Taylor et al., 2013.

Table 2. Needs in Individuals Within One Year of Treatment

Need	% Unmet
Leisure space and activities in hospital	61.9
Age-appropriate hospital care	57.1
Help dealing with boredom	47.6
Help finding meaning of experience	47.6
Access to better food in hospital	42.9
Guidance about future study or career	42.9
Feeling in control over life and decisions	38.1
Information about what happens after treatment	38.1
Complete and honest information about long-term impact of treatment	38.1
Help dealing with overprotective parent/carer	38.1

Note. Based on information from Millar et al., 2010.

Table 3. Needs in Individuals One to Five Years After Treatment

Need	% Unmet
Help focusing on tasks and/or memory	36.4
Information about what happens after treatment	31.8
Help dealing with frustration	31.8
Information about feelings caused by cancer experience	31.8
Approachable healthcare providers	31.8
Help with unwanted thoughts, emotions, and images of cancer	27.3
Complete and honest information about having children	27.3
Help dealing with changes to who I am	27.3
Help dealing with overprotective parent/carer	27.3
Information about support services and available help	27.3

Note. Based on information from Millar et al., 2010.

Table 4. Needs in Individuals Five or More Years Since Treatment	
Need	**% Unmet**
Help focusing on tasks and/or memory	40
To find enjoyment in my life	30
Help dealing with changes to who I am	30
Help coping with loss of independence	30
Help coping with being unable to do the same things as others my age	30
Help thinking about the future	30
Assistance in getting back to work	25
Guidance about future study or career	25
Help dealing with loneliness	25
Help dealing with the possibility of cancer recurrence	25
Note. Based on information from Millar et al., 2010.	

References

Abramson Cancer Center of the University of Pennsylvania. (2012, March 14). Did you know . . . the facts about young adults and cancer? Retrieved from http://www.oncolink.org/coping/article1.cfm?id=1031

Bleyer, A., O'Leary, M., Barr, R., & Ries, L.A.G. (Eds.). (2006). *Cancer epidemiology in older adolescents and young adults 15 to 29 years of age, including SEER incidence and survival: 1975–2000* [NIH Pub. No. 06-5767]. Bethesda, MD: National Cancer Institute.

Canadian Cancer Society Steering Committee. (2009). *Canadian cancer statistics 2009*. Toronto, Ontario, Canada: Canadian Cancer Society.

Millar, B., Patterson, P., & Desille, N. (2010). Emerging adulthood and cancer: How unmet needs vary with time-since-treatment. *Palliative and Supportive Care, 8,* 151–158. doi:10.1017/S1478951509990903

Taylor, R., Pearce, S., Gibson, F., Fern, L., & Whelan, J. (2013). Developing a conceptual model of teenage and young adult experiences of cancer through meta-synthesis. *International Journal of Nursing Studies, 50,* 832–846. doi:10.1016/j.ijnurstu.2012.09.011

SECTION I. Being Sick

Chapter 2. Treatment Decision Making and Dealing With Medical Professionals

Chapter 3. Emotional Effects

Chapter 4. Health Behaviors and Surveillance

Chapter 5. Fertility and Contraception

Chapter 6. Metastatic Disease and Palliative Care

Treatment Decision Making and Dealing With Medical Professionals

A t some points in your cancer experience, you will be asked or encouraged to make a treatment decision or a choice between one or more treatments. You may have already done this—or may have felt annoyed that you weren't given a choice about a treatment you've already had. In the past 20 years, patients have had more choices about their treatment options. The first changes in this regard occurred in the surgical treatment of breast cancer. Studies showed that a lumpectomy (removing the breast lump only) with radiation was as effective as the traditional—and more radical—mastectomy (complete removal of the breast) for many women. This caused a shift from a very patriarchal and patronizing medical system where "the doctor knows best" to one where treatment decisions are made based, in part, on patient preference. This shift also led to an increased need for patients to receive information that is easy to understand and to empower patients to advocate for themselves in a complex medical environment.

[They] told me I had cancer. It sucked. That's all I can really say. I couldn't really express how I was feeling. I basically went numb. And I ended up watching everybody I care about break down, which caused me to become even more numb.

—Daylan, B-cell leukemia

We've come a long way since those early days. For many, it is assumed that they will have a say in their treatment plan, and many patients now have access to the same information as healthcare providers thanks to the Internet, medical libraries and databases, and online advocacy groups. Where do you fall on the spectrum of involvement in treatment decisions? How much do you want to participate in choosing a treatment, and what has your experience been in the past?

What Should I Do?
Preferences for Decision Making

Much research has looked at how patients feel about treatment decision making and what role they want to play in the process. The three kinds of treatment decision making are *active*, *shared*, and *passive*.

- *Active decision making* involves the patient taking the lead in decision making about treatment. This is not seen very often, probably because most of the research on decision making has been done with older people. However, young adults may want to, and probably do, play this kind of role.
- *Shared or collaborative decision making* involves the patient working with the physician to make a treatment decision. In its purest form, the decision is not only made together, but the treatment also is performed collaboratively. This is seen

in chronic disease management (such as in diabetes management, where patients have significant control over what they eat) much more than in cancer treatment, where much of the treatment (surgery, radiation, and chemotherapy) cannot be done by the patients themselves. However, shared decision making about what treatment the patient will receive is fairly common in cancer.

- *Passive decision making* happens when the patient defers to the advice of the physician. This occurs in many instances, as older patients may be socialized to believe that the doctor knows what is best for them, so they don't question or even think that they could be more actively involved. But passive decision making is also seen in people with hematologic cancers (for example, leukemia) where treatment must be started urgently and the treatment regimen is complex.

Not all healthcare providers are comfortable with shared or active decision making. As with any kind of change, some people have to be dragged kicking and screaming toward a new way of doing things. As you can imagine, it is easier for doctors to tell patients what to do and for patients to follow their instructions. But this leads to dissatisfied patients who may fight back by not following those instructions. This then leads them to be labeled as "noncompliant"—a very judgmental and patronizing term—and a vicious circle ensues with no good outcomes for anyone.

If you are not offered the chance to be involved in making decisions about your treatment, ask why not. Even if there are no choices to be made, you should still have as much information as you need to understand why that is so and what is involved in every aspect of your treatment. Later in this chapter we'll discuss communication with healthcare providers and present some tips and strategies to get the most out of your appointments.

It is not always easy for healthcare providers to know what or how much to tell patients unless they say what they want and need at the outset. And of course, patients can and often do change their minds about what they want to know. Some people want to know up front what their prognosis is and how much time they may have. Despite the wide margin of error (in both directions) in predicting how long someone has to live or how a person will react to any given treatment, people often want this information because they have decisions to make about many things in their lives. Some people prefer not to know all the details because they want to maintain hope, and they think that knowing all the bad stuff may take away that hope. There is no right or wrong in this; everyone is different. You can always change your mind and get information that you didn't want originally. However, going the other way is not possible; once you know something, it is a reality for you. But you can change your mind about the amount of information received in the future.

Decision Making Under Difficult Circumstances

Getting a cancer diagnosis is never easy, period. We know that after people hear the words "You have cancer," they only hear about 10% of what they are told after that—and they are often told *a lot* of information. So if they hear only 10% of what comes next, they are going to have a difficult time making sense of it all and making decisions about what comes next. Sometimes treatment has to start immediately or soon, and the patient does not have a lot of time to think about what to do or to consider different options. Or, there may not be any options. And for some people, the shock of the diagnosis leaves them in such confusion that they prefer someone tell them what to do—in other words, passive decision making.

I went through the standard [treatments] . . . at the time there wasn't really any question about what treatment I was going to get. I mean, I guess if I had some markers that are hard to treat, they might have done things differently.
—*Stuart, acute lymphoblastic leukemia*

A number of studies of people with hematologic cancer suggest that they prefer a passive approach to decision making (Carey et al., 2012; Ernst et al., 2010, 2011). It may be that these patients feel overwhelmed by the amount of information and the high-stakes nature of the cancer, and letting the physician make the decisions is the best way to go. In one study, some women with ovarian cancer have reported feeling so traumatized by the diagnosis that they were unable to gather the necessary information to make a decision themselves and left it to their oncologist (Ziebland, Evans, & McPherson, 2006). For some cancers, there are no real decisions to be made. The treatment protocols may not offer any choices and might need to be started right away with no time for reflection or delay.

Woulda-Shoulda-Coulda: Decisional Regret

Making decisions, especially about your health or life, is not easy. When you make a decision and it does not turn out well, or you have unexpected complications or side effects, you may regret that decision. Or perhaps you left it up to someone else—your oncologist or your partner or your parents—and when things did not go well, you got angry or wished that you had played a more active role in the decision. This is called *decisional regret.*

One way to avoid this regret is to be more active in making decisions, such as in shared decision making or maybe even active decision making as described earlier. However, you can still feel regret if you think that, in hindsight, you may have done better if you had chosen something else. It really is a mind game in that you have to try to keep your doubts under control if things don't go well or if you think that you could have done things another way. You will read about ways to reduce anxiety in Chapter 3. Strategies are available to help you focus and bring your mind back from fruitless thoughts about "woulda-shoulda-coulda."

Fighting Back: Empowerment

Empowerment is a word that carries a lot of weight. People who are empowered have some control or mastery over their life, or perhaps just some parts of their life. But for most people, this didn't happen by itself—they had to do something to get that control or mastery. It has been suggested that by being empowered, you can get what you want from a situation. But does that apply to having cancer? There is not much evidence that being empowered helps with getting through the cancer experience. One study (Bulsara, Ward, & Joske, 2004) looked at this in people with hematologic cancer and found that empowerment happened when three conditions were met:

- Having a fighting spirit and determination to cope with the illness
- Being reliant on others within a supportive system including family, friends, and healthcare providers

- Accepting the illness and learning how to manage by finding balance and creating boundaries.

Empowerment also has something to do with what you know. Initially an imbalance exists between the person with cancer and members of the healthcare team. This imbalance centers mainly on knowledge and information. But if both parties share their knowledge, that imbalance goes away (theoretically). They know much more than you do about the disease, but you know more about yourself than they do. They have a duty and responsibility to share their knowledge with you through information sharing. You have a duty to yourself to learn as much about the disease as you can and want to—and you need to share your need for information with the healthcare team in order to create a balance. If either side doesn't play their part, then both are at a disadvantage: your healthcare team won't have an informed and active participant in their treatment plan, and you won't have an understanding care team who can meet your needs. Your ability to share with them depends partly on your ability to communicate with them. So let's talk about communication with your healthcare providers.

Talking the Talk

All communication takes place within a context. For your oncologist, the context is usually a busy clinic with many patients and a pager that goes off every few minutes. For you, the context might be stress related to your diagnosis or treatment or having to wait more than an hour to see your oncologist or nurse. You each bring your own values, beliefs, attitudes, and knowledge to your appointment. And you each have goals for that appointment. For you, the goal might be to get relief for a painful symptom, whereas for the oncologist or nurse, the goal might be to get information from you in order to figure out what is causing the pain. There is similarity, but the goals are different. To achieve these goals, you have to communicate with each other—and that is often where problems begin.

Communication is a two-way street with a giant speed bump in the middle. You talk and the oncologist or nurse listens, and then the oncologist or nurse talks to you (or *at* you in some instances) and you listen as best you can. The listening part is open to interpretation, which is often where the speaker's message gets messed up (the speed bump).

Your listening and interpretation are influenced by anxiety or hope, your ability to understand medical terminology, the amount of sleep you had the night before, your previous experiences with this particular healthcare provider or other healthcare providers, your age, and how you are feeling in the moment, among other factors. Your healthcare providers' ability to hear you is influenced by the amount of sleep they had the night before, whether they've had a break or something to eat, their desire to help you, their confidence in what they know and can do to help you, their emotional connection with you, and their history with other patients like you, among other factors as well. And all of this happens within a context that can make the two-way street like a road race.

Many healthcare providers run very busy clinics, often evident by the number of people you see sitting in the waiting room. They may have allotted just 10 minutes for each appointment, but you might have a long list of things you want to talk about. You know how busy they are, so you try to talk as fast as you can—but your list of what you want to know often doesn't mesh with what your oncologist wants to accomplish in the 10-minute appointment! In addition, some healthcare providers talk in medico-speak, a language that is something like English but with lots of medical terms, often based in Latin, thrown in. Although most medical schools today teach communication skills, those classes fade into the past quite quickly, and older healthcare providers may not have even been taught that stuff. If you are lucky and have doctors or nurses who are really good communicators who take the time to explain things well and make sure that you understand what is happening, hang on to them!

So how can you make yourself heard and listened to? You have to learn how to *ask questions, seek clarification,* and *understand medical language.* First, remember that your healthcare team works for *you.* You can (usually) find another doctor or nurse or radiation therapist. Health care is competitive, especially in the United States and even in Canada. They have a duty and, in most instances, a genuine desire to care for you and give you the best possible chance of remission, cure, or palliation.

The 411 on Asking Questions

- Write down your questions *before* your appointment; having a list will help keep you focused.
- Tell your healthcare providers that you have questions you want to ask; this will alert them to save some time for your questions.
- Offer to come back at another time so that you have enough time to get your questions answered.
- Ask if you can email your questions and get a written reply.
- Wait for healthcare providers to finish a sentence before jumping in with a question.
- Keep asking until you get the answers that you are seeking.

How do you even imagine [or] begin to understand what chemotherapy is going to feel like, much less los-

ing part of your femininity and your body . . . and
then having to have so many surgeries and trying to
make sense of all that, and what it's going to feel like
and how you're going to look.

—*Allison, breast cancer*

Remember that communication is a two-way street. If you feel like you are not getting the answers you want or you are not sure that you understand what you've been told, ask for clarification. The best way to do this is to paraphrase what you've just been told. For example, saying something like "What I just heard you say is . . ." allows the other person to hear what you heard and correct any misunderstandings of what they told you. You can also ask for more information—"Can you please explain that further?"—or ask for more information by saying, "What would happen if . . . ?"

Doctors and nurses have been trained to talk in medical language and shorthand. Some of them are so used to talking like this that they forget that you don't speak the same language. Asking for clarification should help them to understand that you're not quite getting what they're talking about. It also helps if you do some homework and dip your toes into medicospeak. Your doctor might tell you that a test was *negative*—this is not bad; it just means they didn't find something wrong in the test. But if they tell you a test was *positive*, it means that they found something, and that is usually not good. This can be confusing, especially if you are anxious or not feeling well or if you've taken pain medication that makes your head feel spacey. You can (and should) ask for copies of all your tests. You can go over these with your primary care provider or a friend who knows about these things. You can also use the results to track your progress and to better understand what is happening in your body.

Some websites are available that can help you figure out what your healthcare team is talking about, and most libraries have medical dictionaries in their reference section.

These websites can help with medico-speak:

- MedLine Plus medical dictionary from the National Institutes of Health and the National Library of Medicine: www.nlm.nih.gov/medlineplus/mplusdictionary.html
- Webster's New World Medical Dictionary: www.medterms.com/script/main/hp.asp
- A well-known medical dictionary for healthcare providers: http://medical-dictionary.thefreedictionary.com

Getting the Help You Need

The surgeon gave me the results. And said that, because of what it looked like on the ultrasound, it's an indication that it needs to be removed. Well, that's all I wanted to hear. I wanted it gone, whatever it was. Still not even thinking all the way down the road. So, I had a lumpectomy. Didn't ever bother to research any kind of surgery options. I just wanted it gone.

—*Aimee, breast cancer*

Many people with cancer want to find out more about treatment options, clinical trials, the best doctor to treat their cancer, alternative and complementary therapies, and support services. There are thousands of websites where you can find this information, but not all are created equal. You have to be critical and discerning in the maze of self-help and self-promotion out there. Here are some questions to help you figure out if a site is legitimate.

The 411 on Websites

- Is the site associated with a trustworthy organization?
- Does the site recommend a specific treatment, and does it provide information about the pros and cons of that treatment?
- Are there links to references for the claims made on the site? Do these links work?
- Do other legitimate organizations link to this site?
- Is the site sponsored by a for-profit company (look at the section "About Us")?
- Is there a date showing when the site was last updated?
- If this is a personal site, is the person a professional or expert in the content?
- Think about the answers to these questions. Be careful of websites promoting treatments and asking you for money; this is usually a sign that they are not reliable and mostly just want to get you to open your wallet. Compare the information on these sites to what you have been told by your healthcare team; if there is a big difference, trust your healthcare team!

The following are some reliable websites written by healthcare professionals.

- **American Congress of Obstetricians and Gynecologists:** www.acog.org/For_Patients
- **OncoLink (Abramson Cancer Center of the University of Pennsylvania):** www.oncolink.org
- **WebMD:** www.webmd.com
- **National Institutes of Health:** www.nih.gov
- **Mayo Clinic:** www.mayoclinic.com
- **MedicineNet:** www.medicinenet.com
- **Medscape:** www.medscape.com

I think because things happened so quickly . . . I didn't really have a whole lot of time to process it. So the fact that when I was asking him questions, [he was] kind of putting me off a bit . . . it was really frustrating because I wanted to be like, "OK, well, what about this, what about that?" And as soon as I came back from that appointment, he said, "Well, you're going to have this biopsy and stuff." So I started doing all kind of research on how people deal with this. They recommended getting a long list of questions to ask your doctor and all these kinds of things. So I had this huge list of questions to ask. And then when I went to ask him, he was just kind of like, "Oh, don't worry about it; it won't be a problem. We'll just . . . you know, it's just a little thing. We'll do a biopsy and it'll be fine. We'll get it all, and it'll be fine."

—*Robyn, cervical cancer*

Blogs

Many online blogs exist, and some of you may have your own or are thinking about creating one. Blogs are essentially personal reflections on experience. While they serve many real and valuable purposes (such as sharing, support, and information), they are personal and anecdotal and NOT predictive of what you may go through or feel about your own experience with cancer. In short, read with caution and don't believe everything you read. In particular, be very careful about bloggers telling you that product X or Y cured them or prevented them from needing medical treatment. Always do your own research about what you read in blogs and tell your oncology care team about what you are reading; they can help you check out experimental or alternative treatments.

On the positive side, the Internet, blogs, and online support groups can be a lifeline for people with cancer who feel isolated or alone by virtue of where they live, the rarity of their cancer, or their ability to access in-person support and resources. You can connect with and learn from bloggers and in turn create your own blog and reach out to others in this cancer community that you belong to. Just be careful about what and how you share so that you don't preach or mislead or make promises.

Getting a Second Opinion

Many people are nervous about getting a second opinion. They don't want to hurt their doctor's feelings or are scared that the doctor will be mad at them. But you have every right to get a second (or even third) opinion. Most insurance companies will pay for a second opinion because it might save them some money if the first doctor was wrong. You can and should ask your doctors about where to go for a second opinion. If they get defensive, you may want to think twice about staying with them, because they are likely to be defensive with other questions, too.

> So I didn't really feel like I had any options. I've since talked to women who have been in the same position as me and decided not to have a hysterectomy. One [is a] woman in Vancouver who I was set up with as a Cancer Connections [peer supporter] through the Canadian Cancer Society. And she's had the same cancer, same stage, same everything and decided not to have a hysterectomy and she's fine. But I was scared and they said I needed to do it.
> —Robyn, cervical cancer

From Whom Should You Get a Second Opinion?
- Someone who is a specialist and has more qualifications than your first doctor

- Someone who works for a larger cancer center with a bigger volume of patients
- Someone who works at an academic center or hospital
- Someone who has treated someone you know and has been good (as long as he or she is a specialist in your kind of cancer)
- Check out who is publishing in the medical literature about your kind of cancer (search in Google Scholar) and ask if they will see you for a second opinion.

You should never worry about hurting someone's feelings while you are trying to get the best care possible. Ask yourself a simple question: Will I feel better about myself if I try to protect someone else's feelings? The answer is probably "no," so advocate for yourself and get the help you need.

Other Help

Many cancer centers have navigators whose job is to help patients, especially those who are newly diagnosed, navigate the system. They are often registered nurses who know about your kind of cancer. Ask if the cancer center or hospital has a navigation program and if you can be connected to one of the navigators.

Be nice to the reception staff at your doctor's office or clinic. They usually work under a great deal of stress and are used to getting yelled at. When someone is nice to them, they are often inclined to make you a "favorite patient," and that can come in handy.

Most hospitals and cancer centers have patient representatives, or *ombudsmen*, to help patients and their families deal with staff when things go wrong. Most patient complaints are about poor communication. These representatives are experts in getting problems solved before they become lawsuits. They are there to support you as the consumer and can be very helpful when problems arise. Just because they work for the hospital doesn't mean that they will take the side of the hospital or healthcare provider. If you don't like the help you are getting, ask to speak to a supervisor and keep going up the chain until you feel heard. Of course, you also have to be reasonable in what you want and you can't expect miracles, but you can expect to have your questions answered and your complaints heard.

What Comes Next?

Once you've decided on a treatment, or gotten used to the idea that you need treatment, you have to continue to be an advocate for yourself and report what you are feeling and experiencing to your healthcare team. The next chapter will describe how to be on the lookout for symptoms that may need attention from your doctor and nurse outside of usual care. There will also be information about how to take care of yourself during and after treatment.

References

Bulsara, C., Ward, A., & Joske, D. (2004). Haematological cancer patients: Achieving a sense of empowerment by use of strategies to control illness. *Journal of Clinical Nursing, 13,* 251–258. doi:10.1046/j.1365 -2702.2003.00886.x

Carey, M., Anderson, A., Sanson-Fisher, R., Lynagh, M., Paul, C., & Tzelepis, F. (2012). How well are we meeting haematological cancer survivors' preferences for involvement in treatment decision making? *Patient Education and Counseling, 88,* 87–92. doi:10.1016/j.pec.2011.12.014

Ernst, J., Brähler, E., Aldaoud, A., Schwarzer, A., Niederwieser, D., Mantovani-Löffler, L., & Schröder, C. (2010). Desired and perceived participation in medical decision-making in patients with haemato-oncological diseases. *Leukemia Research, 34,* 390–392. doi:10.1016/j.leukres.2009.06.024

Ernst, J., Kuhnt, S., Schwarzer, A., Aldaoud, A., Niederwieser, D., Mantovani-Löffler, L., ... Schröder, C. (2011). The desire for shared decision making among patients with solid and hematological cancer. *Psycho-Oncology, 20,* 186–193. doi:10.1002/pon.1723

Ziebland, S., Evans, J., & McPherson, A. (2006). The choice is yours? How women with ovarian cancer make sense of treatment choices. *Patient Education and Counseling, 62,* 361–367. doi:10.1016/j.pec.2006.06.014

CHAPTER 3

Emotional Effects

M uch of what we read about cancer is framed in a positive way—people "win the battle" and "overcome the odds." A lot is written about surviving and thriving and making the best of a bad situation. What is not talked about much is the struggle that many people go through, the darker side of cancer where depression and anxiety threaten to take over. Oncology care providers are doing a better job of addressing these issues for the most part. Many regularly ask their patients how they are doing, *really* doing, and look for signs that things are not going well, even when the person answers that everything is "fine." Screening for distress is the standard of care in many cancer practices and, beginning in 2015, will be a requirement for all cancer centers and providers in the United States. But what do we mean by "distress"? And how do you know if you are distressed, depressed, or anxious—or all three?

Defining Distress

What is distress? How do you know if you're experiencing it? *Distress* is defined in the dictionary as "pain or suffering affecting the body, a bodily part, or the mind." It is often experienced by people with cancer in the form of depression or anxiety related to fear of recurrence or of developing a secondary cancer and the management of treatment effects such as pain and fatigue. Many of these fears are very real, and the resulting suffering causes significant problems in everyday quality of life.

Research shows that young adults with cancer experience high levels of distress. In one study, 26% reported feeling hopeless, 39% felt sad, and 56% experienced anxiety (Harding, 2012). Young adults with cancer have a lot to lose: as previously discussed in this book, young adulthood is a time where there are many milestones to accomplish (college, work, relationships), and cancer potentially delays or prevents these from being achieved.

> I found that sometimes I would just get so overwhelmed with emotion that I couldn't share it with [my husband]. And that's all he could see, me crying, getting upset . . . "What's wrong? What?" And it's just the overwhelming emotion . . . I have no control. I can't control this. There's nothing I can do. I'm at the mercy of this disease. Sure, I'll bombard my body with all these drugs and chemicals in a hope that it's going to go away. And what if it doesn't?
>
> —Serena, non-Hodgkin lymphoma

Distress is often first seen before treatment starts and is highest one to two years after diagnosis (Yanez, Garcia, Victorson, & Salsman, 2013). This period is described as the *reentry phase,* when survivors try to get back to their usual life and the effects of the cancer and its treatment and the impact on daily life are most noticeable. In the year after treatment, late and long-term effects are at their worst, and alterations in physical, social, and emotional functioning come to the forefront. The active treatment phase is over, and what is left is the new reality of life after cancer. It's no wonder that people get depressed or anxious. The good news is that by the fifth year after diagnosis, cancer survivors have levels of depression and anxiety that are the same as the general population, or even less! So what contributes to distress?

Fear of Recurrence

It's the fear. It's the lack of certainty. It's the lack of control. That's the hardest part because you feel as if cancer always dictates your life. . . . In my case, I now have no breasts. I unfortunately had a situation where the implant damaged my rib. It broke my rib on the right side. And because I'm such a thin woman, I have a lot of concaveness to my right breast. And so every day you're reminded of what cancer has done to you from a cosmetic perspective. Of course, your hair grows back, but there's always that fear, lack of control, and uncertainty that you face on a daily basis if any ache or pain comes your way. I always wonder, when is the shoe going to drop? It doesn't matter if you're [a] recurrent, metastatic, or newly diagnosed patient. We always fear what cancer can do. Is it going to come back, and what will it do to us?

—Kim, metastatic breast cancer

Almost half of all people with cancer experience moderate to high levels of fear of recurrence; most cancer survivors experience this at one time or another. Many describe this fear as like having the sword of Damocles hanging over their head for the rest of their life. This fear of recurrence has lasting implications: quality of life is decreased, emotional coping is reduced, and physical as well as emotional stress responses are common. Young women experience the highest levels of this fear, likely because many young women have young children and the fear of recurrence is intimately linked with their role as caregivers to their families. Put simply, the more you think you have to lose, the greater your fear of losing it all.

> *I think that my biggest loss was just like that subconscious denial of death, that bad things happen to other people . . . . I felt like I was always waiting for the other shoe to drop, and I was sitting under a sneaker tree in a strong wind. It wasn't that I was necessarily afraid that the cancer would come back or that they hadn't gotten it all. I think certainly that was part of it because that's always a concern, . . . but it became like this all-encompassing fear of everything, just not knowing what the next bad thing was going to be. And I found myself having anxiety attacks for a bit. They wouldn't necessarily be triggered by any sort of conscious thought process or anything. I'd just be out doing whatever and just suddenly have this really bad panic attack.*
>
> —Cheryl, cervical cancer

Fear of recurrence is influenced by
- The perception of personal risk, which is related to the type, · grade, and stage of cancer, and treatment
- Anxiety and how well a person copes (or doesn't cope)
- The consequences of the cancer in terms of physical, emotional, and social outcomes

- How intrusive the cancer is in the person's life and how it affects roles and responsibilities in daily life and life goals.

It was my first follow-up and I didn't really know what to expect. I was an absolute mess. I didn't sleep the night before, and I was unbelievably stressed out. I had somehow "psychosomatized" myself into starting to have all of these symptoms that I had had the first time, with the exception of the gaining weight, so I had almost this morbid anticipation of being told that the cancer is back.

—Alison D., kidney cancer

Even for those who are coping well with treatment or life after treatment, triggers may bring back memories of physical pain and suffering or negative emotions. These may include going back to the cancer center or doctor's office for follow-up visits, the smell of the clinic or hospital where you were treated, reading about cancer in books, magazines, or newspapers, hearing about someone else being diagnosed, and having blood drawn, even if the tests are not related to the cancer.

Uncertainty and Cancer

Before the future used to be scary because I didn't know what was going to happen and it wasn't really in my hands. No, it was in my hands. And then I said something like, "Now my life is sort of in God's hands and I trust. I trust that you're going to take care of me." It was just different. Before you're diagnosed, you have your path; you know where you're going in life. Or at least you think you know where

you're going. And then something interrupts that,
and for me, it was the cancer. And my path is sort of
completely erased and washed away. I still don't know
what the future holds. I have no idea.
— *Jennifer, acute myeloid leukemia*

An important aspect of this fear of recurrence is the uncertainty associated with cancer. As many young adult survivors recall, their initial symptoms were often ignored by healthcare providers because young adults "don't get cancer." If you feel that something is wrong with your body or health and you are told that you're fine and that it is not something serious, how much will you trust the rest of what healthcare providers tell you? The experience of cancer is in many ways uncertain all along the disease journey. You don't know how you'll react to the treatments you receive, you don't know how long the side effects may last, and ultimately, you don't know if the treatments will help and if you'll survive.

Anxiety: The Root of Many Problems

Anxiety is a central emotion that many people experience. It can start even before cancer is diagnosed when you realize that something is wrong. After that, your days are filled with waiting for appointments, physical examinations, blood draws, and other tests that may be painful or intrusive. And then you hear the words "you have cancer," and everything changes. Your anxiety now flows from the unknown of cancer treatment, survival statistics, and worry about multiple issues (your family, your job, your education). However, anxiety can be a powerful motivator to make you stick with treatments that before cancer you would never have endured (Traeger, Greer, Fernandez-Robles, Temel, & Pirl, 2012).

> *I'm always carrying it around. I could get sick any time. And there's a better than average chance I will die if I get sick again. Relapsing twice from acute leukemia after having the stem cell transplant . . . it's very bad. Very, very bad, right? But at the same time, like it's not, you know, I'm not paralyzed by anxiety about it. It's just kind of an awareness. I don't think about myself as like 70 or whatever, you know.*
> *—Stuart, acute lymphoblastic leukemia*

The consequences of anxiety, particularly anxiety that does not lessen over time and becomes overriding, are significant. They include

- Inability to make decisions
- Increased physical symptoms
- Disruptions in treatment
- Poor quality of life
- Avoidance of physical activity (because the physical effects, such as increased heart and breathing rate, feel like anxiety)
- Panic attacks.

> *I had a lot of fears, anxieties. I was feeling really depressed. I'd even had some self-harm thoughts and some slightly suicidal thoughts that I had never acted on, but I could tell that I needed some help, that I needed someone to talk to. And I told that to my internist on several occasions and the whole 10 months or so that I was in his care, he was never able to get me in to see anybody, which was really*

the most disappointing and scary part of the whole thing—that I felt like I was in a very, very vulnerable state and it could have been really bad, and no one was helping me. In that sense, dealing with the emotional, spiritual, mental side of what I was going through—I was getting good medical care and attention, but so much time passed in between seeing my doctors and they were never able to refer me to anybody.

—*Naomi, Hodgkin lymphoma*

Many factors contribute to a state of anxiety, but it is important to remember that not everyone with cancer will experience significant anxiety. It is more likely to happen to people who have anxiety issues *before* the diagnosis of cancer. So what factors contribute to anxiety?

- A pre-cancer history of anxiety or trauma
- Avoidant coping styles
- Social isolation
- Being a caregiver to your own children or other members of your family
- Cancer treatments and procedures (such as blood tests)
- Uncertainty and suffering
- Some medications that cause a fast heart rate or shortness of breath
- Substance withdrawal
- Pain, fatigue, shortness of breath, insomnia, and depression

People with significant anxiety tend to have more problems with their cancer care. If you are anxious about having blood drawn or having other tests and procedures, you may try to avoid them and not show up for appointments because you genuinely feel sick at the thought of having the tests; this can then delay treatment further. If you don't have a strong support network, you may be scared to ask for help and being alone can make you feel even more anxious. If your usual way of coping is to avoid unpleasant things, you may delay tests or discussions about your cancer. Feeling uncertain drives some people to demand extra tests to try to reduce the uncertainty, but this often causes more anxiety and fear.

> *I'm scared of running out of time. Every six months I'm terrified of not being able to sleep for days before going to see my surgeon, just waiting for somebody to tell me that it's back and this time it's worse, and I'll have to have all this other stuff. Or I'm afraid that I'll get to where I want to be mentally and emotionally, and it'll be, "Guess what, you have cancer again!"*
> —*Alison D., kidney cancer*

Post-Traumatic Stress

Some people with cancer experience such distress that they are diagnosed with *post-traumatic stress syndrome* (PTSS), also known as *post-traumatic stress disorder* or *PTSD*. PTSS is seen in people who have gone through a natural or man-made disaster and is well known in post-combat veterans. Unlike witnessing a disaster, though, people with cancer endure repeated stress over a long time, including having painful procedures repeatedly and seeing others suffer. Being connected to other people with cancer also means that you may watch them get sicker and even die.

It is thought that younger people with cancer experience this severe form of stress because the cancer happens at a time when they are very vulnerable. Starting out your independent life, finding someone to share your life with, choosing a career, and finding out who you are as a person are important milestones; the threat of cancer makes achieving these milestones difficult. In one study (Kwak et al., 2013), 44% of young adults showed signs of post-traumatic stress one year after diagnosis and 3% had severe signs. This persisted for even longer for a smaller group, and 29% were diagnosed with PTSS.

> *The worst thing is—and I still deal with it every day—is I have a fear of recurrence. I'll have a little thing on my neck and think, "Oh, it's going to my brain." You just live with this and it can be debilitating. You can just get crippled almost by it. Just worrying that the cancer is spreading to your organs. But you just have to get past that and move on every day.*
> *—Robyn, breast cancer*

Signs of post-traumatic stress include
- Having intrusive memories and nightmares where you relive the trauma
- Avoiding reminders and feelings related to the trauma (*emotional numbing*)
- Being hypervigilant and in a constant state of arousal (fast heart rate and breathing)
- Not being able to sleep.

This is exhausting, and people with post-traumatic stress often find themselves unable to work or attend school. They often avoid going to medical appointments because this can make the stressful feelings worse. They often are unable to process information or make decisions. Even though you may feel you are going crazy, you are NOT crazy. But, it is important to get help because feeling this way and having this much stress can make you physically sick and it can affect your ability to make decisions about your health and treatment.

Post-traumatic stress is usually treated with antidepressants and cognitive behavioral therapy (see the following section for some cautions about the use of medications to treat this). Most of what we know about this condition and its treatment comes from the experience of combat veterans or people who have experienced severe trauma from sexual assault or natural or man-made disasters. It is not clear whether individuals with cancer will respond the same way as others.

The 411 on How to Reduce Distress

One way of reducing stress is to change your mind-set to be more optimistic. This may sound strange, but people who have an optimistic outlook on life tend to be less depressed, anxious, and distressed. It also helps if their partner is optimistic (Gustavsson-Lilius, Julkunen, Keskivaara, Lipsanen, & Hietanen, 2012). Think about it this way: if your partner is hopeful about your future, his or her emotional support will be positive and may help to reduce your anxiety and fears about the future.

I've dealt with suffering and pain a lot in my life. So I can continue on and see the bright side, that maybe I'm going to get better. That after this, I'm going to be able to find my place in the world.

—Daylan, B-cell leukemia

There are other ways to reduce distress and anxiety. These include interventions that help to change your way of thinking (cognitive behavioral therapy), reduce symptoms of anxiety (relaxation and supportive counseling), and lessen uncertainty (education about what to expect). There are also medications such as antidepressants and anti-anxiety treatments.

Cognitive behavioral therapy focuses on rehearsing skills to change negative thought processes and behaviors. An example of this is learning how to switch off the cycle of negative thoughts and fears generated by seeing your doctor or nurse practitioner to receive test results. Instead of starting to think about all the bad things that you might hear, you would employ some positive strategies to shut off the negative thoughts and reframe your anticipation in a more positive, less anxious manner.

Supportive counseling allows you a safe and supportive place to express your fears and concerns and process your cancer experience. Counselors who use this approach employ non-directive strategies to allow you to debrief and integrate what you are going through in a supportive environment where you do not have to protect others' feelings and are free to express yourself. They won't tell you what to do, but they listen and make suggestions about how you can cope with what you have been through.

Relaxation exercises help you to control the physical responses to stress and anxiety through mind-body strategies that help you to relax and avoid physical escalation of sensations that raise anxiety levels. These may include guided imagery, yoga, meditation, deep breathing, and progressive muscle relaxation.

Education about specific cancer treatments can lessen your anxiety and uncertainty about new or unknown procedures. For example, a tour of the chemotherapy treatment room along with education about what to expect can help people who have not started chemotherapy to prepare for their treatments. By seeing the physical space and learning about what to expect, fear of the unknown may be reduced.

Medication can be helpful for some people. Three main types of medication are used.

1. Benzodiazepines can help with acute anxiety or panic. They are short acting and highly addictive and worsen fatigue and problems with concentration. They are also not advised for people who use alcohol.

2. Antidepressants such as selective serotonin reuptake inhibitors (SSRIs) and serotonin-norepinephrine reuptake inhibitors (SNRIs) are used to treat anxiety. These medications are effective but may take two to three weeks before they begin to work. They also have side effects, including sexual side effects, that some people are not willing to endure. Some of these medications interact with certain kinds of chemotherapy, making them less effective. It is very important that your oncologist and pharmacist know all the medications you are taking to avoid interactions.

3. Other medications, including antipsychotics and anticonvulsants, may be used to treat anxiety. However, these are not approved for treatment of anxiety and have not been tested in people with cancer. It has been noted that many cancer survivors are reluctant to take medication for anxiety because it makes them feel like they have somehow failed if they need pharmacologic help. Furthermore, some people do not want to add more medication to an already complex treatment regimen (Traeger et al., 2012).

It's Not All Bad: Coping and Finding Meaning

The only thing that I seem to find that works is to redirect my thoughts. So I'll move on to something new and keep myself occupied. [But] as much as

I want to keep busy, it's hard right now because I'm trying to find the balance in life . . . if I do too much, then I get really, really worried and stressed, and that takes a really negative effect on my mind and my body. So it's hard because I don't want to be doing nothing because then the negative thoughts creep in. It's an interesting battle right now to go through. It's tough.

—Jennifer, acute myeloid leukemia

Many cancer survivors are able to find ways to cope with the anxiety and uncertainty of the cancer experience. In one study of young adults with cancer (Trevino et al., 2012), researchers observed different ways of coping. These include

- Proactive coping (targets the problem directly and has positive results)
- Support seeking (was associated with greater anxiety in this study)
- Distancing (avoids confronting the problem directly and has potentially negative outcomes)
- Negative expression (reacting in ways that are not helpful; associated with high levels of grief).

Other coping mechanisms observed included venting, denial, and self-blame. These are seen as maladaptive with the possibility of negative outcomes that may lead to more problems rather than reducing distress.

Why I can't I be my old self? I was so happy with my old self. I have to stop living in the past. I have to live with what I have now, embrace it and love it and make a new me that I can love. I'm still in the process. You have to do what you've got to do with what you have now. But you have to learn to love yourself now.

Love your new normal. [I] hate that new normal, but that's what my nurse would say.

—Serena, non-Hodgkin lymphoma

Many individuals with cancer report positive emotional outcomes including finding meaning and purpose in life, learning to have a more positive outlook on life, experiencing an enriched spiritual life and faith base, and having greater appreciation of life, family, and friends. This is called *post-traumatic growth* and is experienced as

• Stronger sense of self
• Greater sense of purpose
• Stronger sense of personal values
• Increased psychological maturity
• Increased empathy for others
• Better interpersonal relationships
• Greater engagement in activities
• Ability to plan for the future
• Awareness of vulnerability coupled with a sense of self-reliance.

So how do you make this happen? Can you make yourself experience post-traumatic growth? The answer to this question is "maybe." Much of this has to do with how you think about things and how you view your experience. Counseling can help with this, particularly if the purpose is to make sense of the cancer experience and view it in a positive way. Cognitive behavioral therapy can help you to reframe your experience and look for the positive (growth) in even the most painful and traumatic events. You do need a skilled counselor or therapist to help you learn this; if your sessions with the counselor consist mostly of you venting about what has happened, this will not help you to grow and see things differently. The same goes for support groups: if you talk only about the negative things and make no attempt to see how it has made you stronger and more able to cope, you may even find yourself becoming depressed or anxious. Also, the experiences of others may trigger negative memories for you.

> *The best thing that I think came out of it was just having a new appreciation for life and not getting so worked up about small things. We all stress about money and stuff like that. But the real small stuff gets overlooked these days, and you just want to get everything out of every day because you don't know. The world is so uncertain. Nobody knows how long they have here. Just try and get as much accomplished in life as you can. I was never afraid of death. I was more concerned about what was going to happen to my wife if I die, who's going to look after her.*
>
> —*Brian, leukemia*

What Comes Next?

Every experience in life has good and bad, and cancer is no exception. As hard as it is to accept a diagnosis and as challenging as cancer treatments are, you can come out the other side stronger and more appreciative of life. But the dark side is also there; distress and anxiety can take over your life. If you don't ask for or get help, they can make your life truly miserable. Help is available. Although your healthcare providers should routinely offer help to all patients at every visit, you may have to ask for it. That can be difficult, but living with depression or anxiety is even more difficult.

References

Gustavsson-Lilius, M., Julkunen, J., Keskivaara, P., Lipsanen, J., & Hietanen, P. (2012). Predictors of distress in cancer patients and their partners: The role of optimism in the sense of coherence construct. *Psychology and Health, 27*, 178–195. doi:10.1080/08870446.2010.484064

Harding, M. (2012). Health-promotion behaviors and psychological distress in cancer survivors [Online exclusive]. *Oncology Nursing Forum, 39*, E132–E140. doi:10.1188/12.ONF.E132-E140

Kwak, M., Zebrack, B.J., Meeske, K.A., Embry, L., Aguilar, C., Block, R., ... Cole, S. (2013). Prevalence and predictors of post-traumatic stress symptoms in adolescent and young adult cancer survivors: A 1-year follow-up study. *Psycho-Oncology, 22*, 1798–1806. doi:10.1002/pon.3217

Traeger, L., Greer, J.A., Fernandez-Robles, C., Temel, J.S., & Pirl, W.F. (2012). Evidence-based treatment of anxiety in patients with cancer. *Journal of Clinical Oncology, 30*, 1197–1205. doi:10.1200/JCO.2011.39.5632

Trevino, K.M., Maciejewski, P.K., Fasciano, K., Greer, J., Partridge, A., Kacel, E.L., ... Prigerson, H.G. (2012). Coping and psychological distress in young adults with advanced cancer. *Journal of Supportive Oncology, 10*, 124–130. doi:10.1016/j.suponc.2011.08.005

Yanez, B., Garcia, S.F., Victorson, D., & Salsman, J.M. (2013). Distress among young adult cancer survivors: A cohort study. *Supportive Care in Cancer.* Advance online publication. doi:10.1007/s00520-013-1793-8

CHAPTER 4

Health Behaviors and Surveillance

The end of active treatment is a time of reentry into normal life for most cancer survivors. It is also a time that has been neglected in the traditional oncology care system, but this is changing. This chapter discusses what you can do about healthy behaviors as well as explaining the survivorship care plan and ongoing surveillance. Once active treatment is over, the long journey of surveillance, or monitoring, begins.

What is your healthcare team looking for? First, they are looking for signs of recurrence. Each kind of cancer will have specific tests and investigations to do this. They are also looking for signs of long-term and late effects. *Long-term effects* are symptoms that started during treatment and continue for months or years after treatment is over. An example of this is bowel problems that start during radiation therapy and then persist because of damage to the intestines or rectum. *Late effects* are those that start months or years after treatment is over, such as heart problems from certain kinds of chemotherapy. In one study, 59.2% of young adult survivors reported at least one late effect from treatment (Absolom et al., 2009) and had used a variety of services to help them to transition out of active care. One of the ways that your doctors will try to deal with these effects is by a process called *surveillance*—careful monitoring of your health for these long-term and late effects as well as encouraging you to live a healthy lifestyle.

Survivorship Care

Once active treatment is over, the long journey of survivorship care begins. Everyone's journey will be different based on the individual's specific diagnosis, the treatments received, and gender and age. It also depends on when you received treatment, where you live, and what your healthcare providers offer in terms of follow-up care for cancer survivors.

Survivorship care has received a lot of attention since 2006 when the Institute of Medicine published a groundbreaking report, *From Cancer Patient to Cancer Survivor: Lost in Transition* (Hewitt, Greenfield, & Stovall, 2006). This report recognized that the period after active treatment is important and unique and that cancer survivors and their families must be informed about what treatment was given and what comes next. This report recommended that all cancer survivors receive a written care plan called a *survivorship care plan*.

Survivorship Care Plan 101

This care plan has eight key components.
1. A treatment summary with details of the kind of cancer and treatments provided
2. Information about what to expect after active treatment is over

3. Guidelines for other members of the healthcare team about signs of recurrence or the development of new cancers

4. A description of long-term and late effects written so that the survivor can understand what to expect

5. Guidance about nutrition, exercise, healthy behaviors, and risk reduction

6. Psychosocial concerns such as depression, anxiety, and sexual and relationship difficulties

7. Information about financial concerns and issues with returning back to work or school

8. Contact information for all members of the healthcare team for future use

Ideally, the survivorship care plan should be created when you start treatment and added to as you progress. In practice, though, it often is created at the end of treatment by someone in your care team or someone in the survivorship program at the institution. You should be given an appointment to meet with a member of the oncology team to go over the document, and you should receive a copy. A copy also should be sent to your primary care provider (nurse practitioner or family physician). Do not assume that this will happen—you may not have a primary care provider, you may have changed providers, or the cancer center may not have the contact information for your provider. Follow up with your cancer care team to be sure.

Some people collect all their test results from diagnosis through treatment and file them neatly in a binder (or throw them into a desk drawer). This is just part of the information that may be helpful for you after treatment. Don't throw them away, but keep them as an addition to the survivorship care plan (which may or may not have a summary of those test results).

If you are not given a survivorship care plan, you should ask about it, or you can create your own (see below). Care plans come in different formats. Some institutions have their own that are created from your electronic medical record. Others use care plans created online. Here are some websites that offer templates for survivorship care plans:

- **LIVESTRONG Care Plan** (www.livestrongcareplan.org): You create your own care plan on this website by inserting details of your cancer.
- **Journey Forward** (www.journeyforward.org): This is intended for your oncology team to complete. The site also has good information for survivors.
- **Prescription for Living** (www.nursingcenter.com/library/static.asp?pageid=721732): Another template for your oncology team to complete.
- **American Society of Clinical Oncology treatment summaries and care plans** (www.cancer.net/survivorship/asco-cancer -treatment-summaries): These are concise treatment summaries but include very little guidance on long-term or late side effects or suggestions for healthy behaviors.

Because the guidelines for both treatment and survivorship care can change, it is a good idea to know where to look to find updated advice. The following websites are reliable and accurate.

- **National Comprehensive Cancer Network:** Evidence-based guidelines for healthcare providers (www.nccn.org) and up-to-date information for survivors (www.nccn.com)
- **Children's Oncology Group:** Guidelines for follow-up care of children and teenagers with cancer (www.survivorshipguide lines.org)

The entry into survivorship care is important on many levels. It can be a time of celebration—Active treatment is over!—but also of anxiety and uncertainty. A study of adolescents and young adults who were transitioning into follow-up care after active treatment found significant anxiety about recurrence, leaving the safety of the acute care system for an unknown system of follow-up care, not knowing whom to talk to about health issues that had begun in treatment and were still there at the end of treatment, as well as issues related to employment and education and altered relationships (Thompson, Palmer, & Dyson, 2009). The researchers had a number of suggestions for how to deal with these concerns, including maintaining a relationship with the oncology care provider (though this may not be possible depending on the institution where you were treated); developing a written transitional care plan; providing education for the survivor about return to work or school; conducting regular assessments of emotional well-being; providing supportive care for concerns about psychosocial issues; completing appropriate surveillance for long-term and late effects as well as for recurrence and secondary cancers; informing on opportunities for engagement with other young survivors; and offering support for vocational opportunities.

> *You can try to live your day, your life, to the fullest, but you're always watched and monitored very closely, which is great. But it's very challenging to live your life to the fullest when you always have [the cancer] haunting you, especially when you're dealing with the cosmetic effects of what it does.*
> —*Kim, metastatic breast cancer*

While a survivorship care plan can tell you where you've been in terms of treatment, what happens next is, in part, dependent on you. The next section of this chapter deals with health behaviors and what you should avoid in order to reduce your risk of another cancer or other complications.

Health Behaviors

Although many long-term and late effects are not under your control, you can take steps to maximize your health. In Chapter 8, we talk about eating well and exercising. Other health behaviors that can help you to maintain your health include not smoking, not drinking alcohol or drinking only in moderation, protecting your skin from the sun, and not using recreational drugs.

What About Smoking?

About 42% of young adult cancer survivors smoke after diagnosis, almost double the number of young adults without a history of cancer (26%). Furthermore, 25% of childhood cancer survivors smoke in their teenage years (Hollen, Hobbie, Donnangelo, Shannon, & Erickson, 2007). This sounds strange—why would you do something that is known to cause cancer after you've been through it already? There are many potential reasons: The stress of having cancer may lead to smoking as a way to reduce this stress. It may be a way of fitting in with peers, or some people may just not think it's important. If you've already had cancer, you've faced the worst, so how bad could it be if you get it again? It is also difficult to quit. Most smokers have to try many times to stop smoking before they succeed. If you live with smokers, it is really hard to quit for both social reasons and also because you are constantly exposed to secondhand smoke. People who drink alcohol regularly are also more likely to continue smoking, although bans on smoking in bars and clubs have helped to lessen this.

There are, of course, many reasons to quit—social, economic, and health. There also are many resources to help smokers quit, including medication, nicotine replacement methods, support groups, and telephone helplines. Although 70%

of smokers in one study said they wanted to quit, less than 5% managed to quit for good. Those are not good statistics!

Resources to Help You Quit

- Support groups and quit lines have been shown to help people quit smoking.
- The American Cancer Society (800-ACS-2345 [800-227-2345] or www.cancer.org) has useful tips and information about quitting.
- The National Cancer Institute has a tobacco quit line at 800-QUIT-NOW (800-784-8669) as well as a website at www .smokcfrcc.gov.

What About Alcohol?

The safety of alcohol consumption for cancer survivors depends on the kind of cancer you have, whether you are a man or woman, and whether you are in active treatment or remission. There has been very little research on alcohol use and cancer survivors, especially young adults, but we do know from one study that 49% of teenage cancer survivors drink alcohol (Hollen et al., 2007). Cancers of the head and neck are associated with the use of alcohol, and continuing to drink may increase the risk of recurrence or development of a second cancer: as few as two drinks a day can increase your risk of a second cancer fourfold. Alcohol is processed through the liver and can cause inflammation of that organ, so drinking during treatment can interfere with the metabolism of chemotherapy agents. And, in turn, chemotherapy and radiation therapy cause inflammation of the liver, so drinking alcohol may causc additional problems for your liver as it tries to metabolize all these substances. Alcohol also can irritate the lining of the mouth and throat and make stomatitis or dry mouth worse. If you have mouth sores, drinking alcohol is going to hurt.

> *I drink more than I should . . . I'm always think-*
> *ing to myself every time I put something negative into*
> *my body, Are you more susceptible to getting an effect*
> *from this? And that's stress on the mind, too. Every-*
> *body I hang around with lives the party life. . . . Ob-*
> *viously I love time with my family, but any time I'm*
> *ever with my friends, they don't live the healthiest life-*
> *styles. They're not the ones at the gym and jogging in*
> *the park.*
>
> —Brian, leukemia

While social drinking is easier to control than smoking, there are often pressures to drink with your friends and family. Alcohol consumption is part of our society: we celebrate with champagne, commiserate over a glass of wine or liquor, and drink beer at a ballgame. It can be really hard to refuse to drink when everyone else is doing it, and others may tease or pressure you to drink just to fit in.

Dealing With Pressure: How to Say "No"

Using humor can help when responding to pressures to drink alcohol:

- "I prefer to get my calories from food, not alcohol."
- "Where I come from, the legal drinking age is 45."
- "My doctor told me that if I drink, my skin will turn orange."

On the other hand, if you do drink, you may find that people are concerned that you are drinking (because of the cancer) and may comment or even take away the bottle or glass. These actions are not necessarily based on knowledge and usually are intended to "help" you. You need to tell people what you are allowed to do and what is recommended. Although it may be irritating to constantly have to talk about this, in the long run you may save yourself from awkward situations.

Dealing With Do-Gooders: "Are You Sure You Should Be Drinking That?"

Try some snappy answers when people get in your face:

- "I ran out of mother's milk, and this was a good substitute."
- "My doctor has prescribed a beer a day to help me get a better attitude."
- "This? Oh, this is only 60 proof—I keep the good stuff for special friends."

Sun Safety

Very little research has been done on sun exposure in cancer survivors. One study showed that sunscreen lowers the risk of skin cancer, the same as in the general population. It is well known that sun exposure is dangerous in terms of skin cancer and that proper protection can help to avoid the development of two of the most common skin cancers, basal cell and squamous cell. While there are no guidelines for sun safety in cancer survivors, follow these common-sense suggestions.

- Avoid direct sun exposure between 10 am and 4 pm, when the sun is hottest
- Cover up with a long-sleeved shirt.
- Wear a hat.
- ALWAYS wear sunscreen on exposed areas.
  - Look for a sunscreen that is labeled *broad spectrum* (protects against both UVA and UVB rays).
  - Use sunscreen that is labeled SPF 30 (any higher provides no extra protection).
  - Apply it thickly—a full palm of sunscreen for your arms, neck, and face, one palmful for your legs, and so on.
  - Reapply every two hours and after swimming, sweating, or wiping off with a towel.

– Check the expiration date on the bottle or tube; most sunscreens expire in two to three years.

There has been a lot of talk in recent years about vitamin D and its role in cancer prevention. A major source of vitamin D is sun exposure. So how can you get this important vitamin without increasing your risk for skin cancer? Actually, you probably get enough sun exposure just going about your daily activities in sunny climates: 10–15 minutes in the sun every day is thought to be sufficient for our vitamin D requirements. That is very different from sunbathing or going to a tanning salon. (Claims about vitamin D from tanning beds are false—the light is not the same as that provided by the sun and is far more dangerous.) For those of us who live in northern geographic areas or rainy places, supplements are advisable, especially during the winter. Vitamin D is stored in the body, and high levels can be toxic; take only the recommended daily dose (400–800 IU). Some doctors recommend that you keep out of the sun entirely and use vitamin D supplements to get your daily requirements. Plus, that way you know how much you are getting, unlike with sun exposure.

What About Recreational Drugs?

Recreational drug use is a touchy subject. This section is not intended to approve or disapprove of or judge those who use recreational drugs. For as long as humankind has existed, people have found ways to use plants, fruits, and vegetables as intoxicants. In the 1930s, alcohol was prohibited in the United States for various reasons, and a thriving illegal trade ensued. Generational differences often exist in attitudes toward recreational drug use, with older generations viewing it negatively (even though they may have tried similar things when they were younger) while younger generations are more in favor of it, in part because youth is a period of exploration. Some people develop their own set of rules regarding drug use; for example, anything natural (marijuana and psychedelic mushrooms) is okay, but anything synthetic (Ecstasy and methamphetamine) is not. Prescription medication may be used or abused recreationally when it is meant to be used to control pain or other symptoms. More about that later.

Very few studies have looked at cancer survivors and the use of recreational drugs. The few that exist studied marijuana. Marijuana has been used for years to treat pain, increase appetite, lift mood, and decrease nausea and vomiting from chemotherapy. The active ingredient in marijuana, delta-9-tetrahydrocannabinol (THC), has been synthesized and is produced in two products that are approved by the U.S. Food and Drug Administration: dronabinol (Marinol®) and nabilone (Cesamet®). Another product, Sativex®, is approved for use in Canada (Engels et al., 2007). These substances are not used as frontline treatment for nausea and vomiting but rather when symptoms have not responded to standard medications (Todaro, 2012).

Many people with cancer obtain marijuana illegally. However, in the United States, 18 states and the District of Columbia have legislation allowing the purchase of medical marijuana (at the time of this writing), and cancer is one of the conditions that qualifies for the use of medical marijuana (National Conference of State Legislatures, 2013). But it still remains a federal offense to possess marijuana (Hoffmann & Weber, 2010). Smoking marijuana allows for rapid absorption (Green & De-Vries, 2010) and often is the preferred method of intake, but marijuana smoke is potentially harmful. It contains most of the same cancer-causing substances as tobacco smoke but at 50% higher concentrations and with three times the level of tar (Bowles, O'Bryant, Camidge, & Jimeno, 2012). In one study, 16% of childhood cancer survivors admitted to using marijuana in their teens (Hollen et al., 2007). This statistic is from an older study and may be higher today.

The recreational use of painkillers (especially narcotics, such as codeine) is of concern in cancer survivors. Cancer itself and certainly its treatments can be painful, and therefore many people with cancer are given pain medication, often narcotics. Some patients fear addiction and do not take prescribed medication and receive inadequate pain control. Others do take pain medication and get relief. However, for most survivors, the need for pain medication goes away over time. Keeping this medication in the home poses risks to family members. Narcotics can be highly addictive and often are abused. These medications need to be kept in a safe place where others are not able to access them. Having them around also can be a temptation to some cancer survivors who may use them to get high or share them with friends. This is dangerous and illegal.

The 411 on Keeping Painkillers (and Other Medications) Safe

- Always keep controlled substances locked up. This includes hydromorphone (Dilaudid®), oxycodone (OxyContin® and Percocet®), and hydrocodone (Vicodin®).
- Antianxiety medication, such alprazolam (Xanax®), also needs to be locked up.
- Keep medications in their original containers so you know what they are.
- Take medications to a pharmacist to be destroyed when they are close to their expiration date or are no longer needed.
- Don't hoard painkillers. If you need them, you can get a refill from your doctor or healthcare provider, who will know what and how much you should be taking.

What Comes Next?

This chapter has dealt with the physical effects of cancer and behavioral and surveillance issues for survivors. Another physical effect of cancer treatment is changes to your ability to have children. The next chapter will deal with fertility issues. Even if having kids is very far off your radar right now, things may change for you. You may want to read this chapter to find out what you can do now or in the future to preserve fertility or how to prevent pregnancy before you're ready to be a parent.

References

Absolom, K., Eiser, C., Michel, G., Walters, S.J., Hancock, B.W., Coleman, R.E., ... Greenfield, D.M. (2009). Follow-up care for cancer survivors: Views of the younger adult. *British Journal of Cancer, 101*, 561–567. doi:10.1038/sj.bjc.6605213

Bowles, D.W., O'Bryant, C.L., Camidge, D.R., & Jimeno, A. (2012). The intersection between cannabis and cancer in the United States. *Critical Reviews in Oncology/Hematology, 83*, 1–10. doi:10.1016/j.critrevonc.2011.09.008

Engels, F.K., de Jong, F.A., Mathijssen, R.H.J., Erkens, J.A., Herings, R.M., & Verweij, J. (2007). Medicinal cannabis in oncology. *European Journal of Cancer, 43*, 2638–2644. doi:10.1016/j.ejca.2007.09.010

Green, A.J., & De-Vries, K. (2010). Cannabis use in palliative care—An examination of the evidence and the implications for nurses. *Journal of Clinical Nursing, 19*, 2454–2462. doi:10.1111/j.1365-2702.2010.03274.x

Hewitt, M., Greenfield, S., & Stovall, E. (Eds.). (2006). *From cancer patient to cancer survivor: Lost in transition.* Washington, DC: National Academies Press. Retrieved from http://iom.edu/Reports/2005/From-Cancer-Patient-to-Cancer-Survivor-Lost-in-Transition.aspx

Hoffmann, D.E., & Weber, E. (2010). Medical marijuana and the law. *New England Journal of Medicine, 362*, 1453–1457. doi:10.1056/NEJMp1000695

Hollen, P.J., Hobbie, W.L., Donnangelo, S.F., Shannon, S., & Erickson, J. (2007). Substance use risk behaviors and decision-making skills among cancer-surviving adolescents. *Journal of Pediatric Oncology Nursing, 24*, 264–273. doi:10.1177/1043454207304910

National Conference of State Legislatures. (2013, August). State medical marijuana laws. Retrieved from http://www.ncsl.org/issues-research/health/state-medical-marijuana-laws.aspx

Thompson, K., Palmer, S., & Dyson, G. (2009). Adolescents and young adults: Issues in transition from active therapy into follow-up care. *European Journal of Oncology Nursing, 13,* 207–212, doi:10.1016/j.ejon.2009.05.001

Todaro, B. (2012). Cannabinoids in the treatment of chemotherapy-induced nausea and vomiting. *Journal of the National Comprehensive Cancer Network, 10,* 487–492. Retrieved from http://www.jnccn.org/content/10/4/487.long

CHAPTER 5

Fertility and Contraception

S ome young adults have far-off, someday plans for parenting; for others, those plans may be closer and more immediate. What effects do cancer and its treatment have on future fertility? And how do you even think about that when newly diagnosed and overwhelmed with information? If you're on the other side of treatment, can you even remember what you were told about it? How do you know if you can or can't get pregnant or get someone pregnant? This chapter will describe the potential effects of cancer treatments on fertility as well as the constantly changing world of fertility preservation. It will also talk about the need for contraception (birth control) and safer sex practices for young adult cancer survivors.

Effects of Cancer Treatment on Fertility

All cancer treatments can affect fertility. Depending on whether you are male or female, different outcomes are possible.

Impact of Surgery

- Surgery to the male pelvis (for colorectal cancer, for example) may damage the two tubes that carry sperm from the testicles (the vas deferens).

- Some surgeries result in semen being pushed into the man's bladder instead of out of the penis (this is called *retrograde ejaculation*). If this happens, the man cannot get his partner pregnant naturally. There are ways to get the sperm out of the bladder, but they involve procedures and aren't exactly romantic!
- If the prostate has been removed, there is no ejaculate, and so pregnancy is not possible without extracting the sperm directly from the testicles.
- Removal of a woman's uterus or ovaries will result in the woman not being able to conceive or carry a fetus, that is, not get pregnant.
- If only the cervix is removed, the woman may be able to get pregnant but may not be able to carry a pregnancy.

Impact of Radiation

- In men, radiation to the testicles can impair their ability to produce sperm and also testosterone. This can lead to infertility, as well as sexual problems because of low testosterone levels (see Chapter 7 on sexuality).
- In women, radiation to the ovaries can result in premature menopause (caused by loss of estrogen, which is produced in the ovaries) and loss of eggs (ovarian reserve). Radiation damage to the uterus itself can result in a shrinking of the uterus that cannot stretch with a growing fetus. Radiation also can damage the lining of the uterus, preventing implantation of a fertilized egg.

Impact of Chemotherapy

Chemotherapy has the potential to affect fertility, but this depends on the kind of chemotherapy and the age of the person when treatment occurs.

- The greatest risk for infertility is for those who have a stem cell transplant with total body irradiation and treatment with cyclophosphamide or busulfan (Salama et al., 2013).

- For women in their 30s with breast cancer, combination chemotherapy with cyclophosphamide, methotrexate, fluorouracil, doxorubicin, and epirubicin poses a slightly lower risk for infertility.
- For some chemotherapy agents, such as taxanes, monoclonal antibodies, and tyrosine kinase inhibitors, we don't know the risks to fertility because many of these medications are relatively new.

Women are born with a finite number of eggs. Therefore, damage to the ovaries may result in permanent infertility. Men, on the other hand, are constantly producing sperm, so they may recover fertility after treatment. Much depends on the type of treatment, the dosage given, the age at which it was given, and what attempts, if any, were made to preserve fertility.

Preserving Fertility

It's more upsetting because we were at that stage in our life where we were prepared to start trying to have a family. And that was immediately stopped. Going into treatment, we knew that the chances of me being able to conceive later on was going to be slim, like 13%, I think it was, because I was going to be going through chemotherapy and total body radiation. However, during the very first treatment round, we were scheduled to go to the fertility clinic to figure out what options we had to preserve some eggs. It turned out that it takes approximately four to six weeks for the procedure to happen. After finding that information out, the doctors looked it over and, because of the stage of my cancer, [determined] I probably would have relapsed in between those weeks. So I didn't real-

> *ly have the ability to do the preservation, which is re-*
> *ally upsetting because they knew how much I wanted*
> *to have children.*
>
> —*Jennifer, acute myeloid leukemia*

Fertility preservation is an area of much research and attention within the oncology community. We will talk about the barriers and facilitators to discussions about this in the following pages. But first, here is what we know about preserving fertility for both men and women. This is an evolving field with advances being made, but also an area of medicine where false hope is possible and promises may not always become reality.

Options for Men

Sperm banking: This is the least invasive of all the procedures and the most established. The man masturbates into a cup, and the semen is sent to a laboratory to be frozen and stored. Semen is usually collected on two to three separate occasions with 24–48 hours between samples. However, if treatment must be started immediately, even one sample is better than none. The sperm remain viable for many years and are thawed when needed. The man's partner either has the semen placed into her uterus near the time that she is ovulating (known as *artificial insemination*) or the sperm is used to fertilize a harvested egg to create an embryo in the laboratory that is later placed into her uterus. Although the process is relatively simple and many men do it, one study showed that of the men who banked sperm, only 7% used it for assisted reproduction (Olatunbosun & Zhu, 2012).

Shielding of the testicles: For men who need radiation to the pelvis, metal shields are used to protect the testicles from radiation damage. This is not 100% effective, and some damage may still occur because of scatter from the radiation.

Testicular tissue banking: This is an experimental procedure to remove and freeze tissue from the testicles that theoretically can be implanted back into the body after treatment is over. It is not known how best to do this, and no live births have occurred from this procedure yet. There is also concern that the tissue may contain cancer cells that would then be reintroduced into the man's body and cause a recurrence or new cancer.

> *The question of if I'm sterile or not, or if I could become sterile, never was asked because I really don't think that could happen, but who knows. So if I were to become sterile now, it would suck if I would ever want a family. But I could always adopt or something.*
>
> —Daylan, B-cell leukemia

Options for Women

The options for women are much more limited.

Embryo banking: This is the only well-established method of preserving fertility. The woman's eggs are fertilized using sperm from her partner or a donor, and embryos are created. These are then frozen and implanted into the woman herself or a surrogate at a later date. One of the biggest challenges with this method is that cancer treatment must be delayed for up to three weeks to allow for stimulation of the ovaries to produce multiple eggs that are then extracted. If the woman's cancer is hormone dependent, this procedure cannot be done because the hormones needed for the stimulation may make the cancer worse. In addition, a male partner who can donate sperm is required, which is a significant barrier for those who do not have a partner. It is also not an appropriate method for girls who have not yet gone through puberty. The live birth rate for embryo freezing is 27% per frozen embryo transfer, less than 1 in 3 chance each time an embryo is implanted. Costs are considerable for all of the procedures, from stimulating the ovaries to creating the embryo and freezing it, as well as thawing and implanting it later. These costs are usually not covered by insurance plans.

Ovarian transposition: This is a surgical procedure to move the ovaries out of the treatment field when radiation is given to the pelvis. It does not delay treatment and is suitable for girls before puberty. However, the success rate for future pregnancies is only about 50%.

Ovarian shielding: External shields can be used to protect the ovaries from radiation damage. This is another established prevention measure for girls or women who need radiation to the pelvis. However, damage can still occur because of scatter of the radiation rays.

Ovarian suppression: This is an experimental although often used practice to try to shut down the ovaries during treatment to protect eggs from the effects of chemotherapy. The success of this method is debatable, and no clear evidence has shown that it is effective in protecting fertility.

Oocyte (egg) preservation: In this experimental procedure, eggs are removed from the ovaries after hormonal stimulation and then frozen. They can later be thawed and fertilized by sperm to create an embryo that is then implanted into the woman or a surrogate. The same cautions that apply to embryo preservation apply to this procedure: it is not suitable for women with hormone-dependent cancers, and it requires a delay in treatment. But it is an option for single women. Although great strides have been made in freezing and thawing eggs, the success rate is still very limited (a live birth rate of only 6% per frozen egg), and the costs are very high.

Ovarian tissue freezing and transplantation: In this experimental treatment, ovarian tissue is surgically removed from the woman and frozen. It is then later transplanted back into her body after treatment, either onto a remaining ovary or close to it (called *orthotopic* site transplantation) or somewhere else in the body (called a *heterotopic* site, such as the forearm) if the woman had received radiation to the pelvis. Orthotopic transplantation has resulted in 15 live births, but no live births have occurred after heterotopic transplantation (Salama et al., 2013). There is significant concern about reintroducing cancer to the woman's body with both of these procedures. The time frame is also very limited for the woman to become pregnant before eggs are lost because of decreased blood supply after transplantation. As you can imagine, this is very expensive and not covered by insurance.

Options available after treatment: Using eggs harvested from a donor that are then fertilized with the male partner's sperm and implanted in the woman has a live birth rate of about 50% per cycle. Obtaining an embryo from another couple may also be a possibility; the success rate of this is not known. Some couples choose to have another woman carry a pregnancy for them, either with a frozen embryo of their own or with one using the surrogate's egg. Legal issues may exist with these options and vary from state to state and country to country.

"What Did They Say?"

What are young adults told about fertility preservation and the potential for fertility loss? Well, that depends. A number of factors influence information sharing about this topic.

They told us about that. It wasn't something at the time that I was too concerned about. Also, things hap-

pened so fast that I don't know if there would have been time to do any banking.

—Graham, leukemia

Age

The age of the person newly diagnosed with cancer makes a big difference not only about *what* but also *whom* is told. If the patient is younger than 18 years old, the topic may be raised with the parents. They may be so shocked by the diagnosis and the threat to their child's life that they can't process the information. They may not be able to see beyond the immediate danger to their child, and childbearing is a far-off and abstract concept. Although parents of underage children and teenagers are legally the guardians and medical decision makers for their child, they may not be able to anticipate what that child or teen will want later in life. They have to make the best decision at the time, which may not be the best decision in the long term for their child.

I definitely brought up questions about fertility at the beginning when I met with my oncologist. They set up an appointment with me for a fertility specialist. That was early on, maybe a month before I started treatment. I've always wanted to have kids, so I was really interested to hear what my options were. I only went one time and I went with a family friend, which I think was smart because if I had gone with my parents, I think I would have been less free to make up my own mind about what was good for me and more swayed by what my parents thought was best for me. So she came in with me, and they sat me down, and the doctor didn't come in right away, but one of her assistants came in and laid out the whole process of freezing eggs and freezing embryos. So we talked about what would be involved in that and what the timeline would be, and she emphasized that it would have to happen very quickly, like within a week or two, to get it all done before I started treatment. They asked questions like, "Are you in a relationship?" and I said, "I'm kind of freshly out of one, but he's still in my life," and she was like, "Would you be in a position to be able to ask him to donate sperm for an embryo?"

—*Naomi, Hodgkin lymphoma*

Gender

Men are told about fertility preservation more often than women. This may be because sperm banking is relatively simple to do, does not delay the start of treatment, and does not involve invasive procedures. In a large Swedish study, 80% of men were told about the impact of their treatment on fertility, 68% were told about sperm banking, and 54% banked sperm. Only 48% of women received information about the impact on fertility, and just 14% were told about fertility preservation. As a result, only 2% underwent fertility preservation (Armuand et al., 2012). In a study from the United Kingdom, men were actively encouraged to bank sperm, while only negative information about fertility preservation was presented to women (Peddie et al., 2012). Women were told that fertility preservation was experimental and had poor outcomes and that the need to start treatment urgently was greater than the need to preserve fertility.

Healthcare Provider

Healthcare provider attitudes play an important role in what is discussed. Participants in some studies stated that their healthcare providers seemed uncomfortable talking about this topic (Niemasik et al., 2012). Others said that their health-care providers wanted to delay talking about fertility until they were older (Gorman, Bailey, Pierce, & Su, 2012), but by then it would be too late!

Not all oncology care providers know the latest evidence about fertility preservation for their patients and therefore do not open the discussion. They may assume that nothing can be done for patients with certain kinds of cancer or of a certain age. Healthcare providers should maintain connections with fertility specialists who do know about the latest methods and who can talk to patients.

Discussion about fertility also may depend on whether the patient already has a child or children. Healthcare providers may assume that if the patient already has one or more children, that should be enough, and fertility preservation is not needed (Niemasik et al., 2012).

This is a complex issue. There is usually a time crunch after a cancer diagnosis—most people want to start treatment as soon as they can, and often their oncology care providers insist on this. So the impact on fertility is not discussed, and fertility preservation is not even mentioned. But it is important information on many levels. Associations for oncology care providers (such as the American Society of Clinical Oncology) have recommendations and guidelines stating that fertility preservation options should be discussed as early as possible when planning treatment to allow for patients to decide what is right for them.

My oncologist did mention it, because I was only 25. She asked me, and I didn't want to even talk about it because it wasn't a consideration for me. So we discussed it, but it wasn't anything. And then I had my ovaries out because of the gene. With the gene, ovari-

an cancer is a high risk . . . So I didn't want to consid-
er having biological children because I had the gene.

—Melinda, breast cancer

Where Are the Patient Voices About Fertility Preservation?

Although thinking about having children is the last thing on some people's minds, some oncology care providers see the offer of fertility preservation as a sign of hope for a life for patients beyond cancer (Crawshaw, Glaser, Hale, & Sloper, 2009). Others find that thinking about fertility is another challenge during a time when major decisions must be made about treatment and a lot of information has to be absorbed and acted on—often in a short period of time. Some women report feeling too overwhelmed and fearful to advocate for themselves or ask for information about the impact of treatment on fertility and options for fertility preservation. Others who were unsure about wanting children in the future were not given any information at all (Niemasik et al., 2012).

> *They didn't really talk about children. My aunt was concerned. She said I may want to consider harvesting my eggs. The only thing is the amount of time involved to harvest the eggs. I was the one who brought up the topic with the doctor, the hematologist. And he said, "I'll look into it." But with these types of drugs, they said there's not a whole lot of concern that it would affect my fertility in the sense that I couldn't get pregnant. It would affect me that it could bring on menopause 10 years earlier than when my mother went through it. So instead of going through meno-*

pause in my mid to late 40s, I could be going through it in my mid to late 30s. So here I am, 23 years old, saying, "OK, here's your 10-, 12-year window to have kids."

—Serena, non-Hodgkin lymphoma

Some women are concerned about the impact of loss of fertility on existing or future relationships. What if your partner doesn't want children, now or in the future, but a decision has to be made in a hurry to bank sperm or freeze eggs? What if you don't attempt fertility preservation and then meet someone who really wants to have children and you can't?

They briefly brought up, "You might want to talk to a lawyer before you decide" because of course if you're producing embryos out of marriage, technically, whose property is that? What rights would the father have, and what rights would the mother have? And responsibilities? Should I decide not to use them, would he be able to use them with someone else? It's very complicated. Very, very emotional. And I found the whole experience kind of traumatic because it came at me all at once, right when I walked in the door. And with the short timeline, I had to make a decision right there and then, basically, because we'd have to start right away. So my initial reaction was, "Oh my God, I don't think I can do this, and I kind of feel like I have to, and I don't know what my chances will be after treatment of being able to have a kid." And then the doctor came in and calmed my fears. She showed me that people in my age group with Hodgkin's lymphoma who have treatment, the risks to fertility are quite low and they have pretty good outcomes with people who try to have kids a reasonable amount of time after. The pressure was still kind of on because she said things like, "You don't want to wait too long; you're 24 now, but you don't want to wait too long before you start trying to have kids." And that was scary because these days people into their 40s are starting to have kids, and I feel like I have to think about it and have kids before I turn 30 because my clock is ticking much faster than most people's.

—Naomi, Hodgkin lymphoma

And what about the risk to your health from delaying treatment long enough to do something to preserve fertility? This can cause stress in a relationship where your partner is worried about losing YOU, and you want to make an embryo and delay treatment? Some young women are worried about their long-term health and whether it's fair to have children after having cancer with the threat of recurrence or a premature death and its impact on young children. Others are worried about the effect of a future pregnancy on their own survival (Gorman et al., 2012).

Cautions and Costs

We've all seen miracle stories on daytime TV of people who were told they would never have children and then have twins or triplets or quadruplets. "Test tube" babies are brought into the studio, tiny and cute, and we think that it's easy and anyone can do it, so why worry now when you can have a miracle child of your own when you're ready? Well, that's TV—it never tells the whole story. Although great strides have been made in the world of new and assisted reproductive technologies, this is a field that in many ways is still in its infancy (poor choice of words, perhaps). Success rates are mostly very low and costs very high.

I'm OK with not having kids. I'm totally at peace with it. But I still struggle with that choice being taken from me. . . . I have a niece who got pregnant, and I struggle with that because she's so young and she was able to just get pregnant, and that if I wanted to have a child, I would have to plan and save and think about it and go out and fill out forms and go through a super-long, intense process, and that part upsets me.

—Melinda, breast cancer

You've read earlier in this chapter of the limited successes from these procedures, ranging from a low of 6% for live births with egg freezing to a high of 27% for embryo freezing. For many people with cancer, cost is also a consideration. Assisted reproductive technologies cost money—a lot of money. Financial assistance for fertility treatment may be available (see the Fertile Hope for U.S. citizens and Fertile Future for Canadians websites discussed later in chapter), but these programs have strict eligibility criteria based on household income, type of cancer and treatment, and other factors.

Also unscrupulous practitioners are out there who can set up a clinic, make promises and quote faborable success rates, and take your money with no responsibility to you, your health, or your well-being. When choosing a fertility specialist, ask for a referral from your oncologist or nurse, preferably at a university- or hospital-affiliated program. These specialists and their clinics will be accredited and should share accurate statistics about success rates before beginning treatment. They will also have support services available such as social workers, counselors, or psychologists to help you with the emotional challenges associated with the procedures and outcomes.

What About Contraception?

It may seem strange to talk about the need for contraception (birth control) after the long and detailed discussion about infertility. But, young adult cancer survivors can and do get pregnant or get their female partner pregnant, and the timing may not always be right. Cancer survivors may overestimate their risk of becoming infertile and may not take the necessary precautions to avoid pregnancy. Young cancer survivors may also feel pressured to have sex if they believe that they have limited time and want to experience life to the fullest. Research suggests that young adults with cancer are as sexually active and interested as their peers without cancer.

The 411 on Contraception for Women

Hormonal Methods

- Oral contraceptives ("The Pill"): combined estrogen and progestin
  - Should not be used by women with a hormone-dependent cancer (such as breast or endometrial)
  - Safe and reliable if used properly
  - Vomiting and mucositis from chemotherapy may reduce effectiveness.
  - Used with caution in patients with thrombocytopenia (low platelets), but continuous cycling with the oral contraceptive pill may help to minimize or stop bleeding
  - May interact with some antibiotics, and some medications reduce effectiveness of the oral contraceptive.
  - Should not be used in bone marrow transplant recipients who are on steroids or cyclosporins to prevent graft-versus-host disease
- Contraceptive patch or vaginal ring
  - Contains estrogen and progestin, but instead of being taken by mouth, it is placed on the skin (patch) or in the vagina (ring)
  - Stays in place for one month and then needs to be replaced (setting a reminder may be helpful)
  - Same cautions for women with a hormone-dependent cancer

- Progestin-only pills
  - Higher failure rate than combination estrogen and progestin pills
  - Not recommended to prevent pregnancy because they require careful and exact timing of use
  - Useful for emergency contraception (also called the "morning-after pill") and used as a backup when unplanned and unprotected intercourse occurs. Does not cause an abortion as is commonly suggested by opponents. Needs to be taken within 48 hours of unprotected intercourse.
- Injectable contraceptive (Depo-Provera®)
  - Effective; provides long-term (12 weeks) protection against pregnancy
  - Should be used with caution in women undergoing chemotherapy because the injection deep into the muscle can cause significant pain and deep bruising
  - Prolonged use can cause decreased bone density.
- Intrauterine device
  - Small wire/plastic device placed in the uterus
  - May cause excessive bleeding and cramping
  - Some devices release progestin slowly, which causes loss of menstruation.
  - May increase the risk of sexually transmitted infections (STIs) or pelvic infection if the woman has multiple partners
  - Not recommended for women during chemotherapy

Barrier Methods

- Female condom: Plastic sheath that is placed into the vagina before intercourse
  - Protects against STIs and is nonhormonal
  - Low acceptance rate leads to high failure rate because it requires consistent use
- Cervical cap or diaphragm: Rubber or latex cup that is placed over the cervix
  - Does not protect against STIs
  - Should be used with spermicidal jelly or foam to increase effectiveness
  - Low acceptance rate leads to high failure rate because it requires consistent use

The 411 on Contraception for Men

The condom is the only available method of male contraception. It is effective if used consistently and correctly.

- Should be used with extra lubricant to prevent breakage
- Needs to be removed after ejaculation to prevent accidental slippage
- Available in many sizes (snug to extra-large) and is cheap and easily available
- Prevents STIs and also protects from exposure to chemicals if used while on chemotherapy

The following methods are NOT effective and have high failure rates:
- Abstinence (because most people find this impossible)
- Withdrawal method
- Periodic abstinence (no sex when the woman is ovulating, also known as *fertility awareness*, *natural family planning*, and the *rhythm method*)

The Low-Down on Sexually Transmitted Infections

People with cancer may be more susceptible to getting an STI than the general public because of immune suppression, and in turn, getting an STI can be more dangerous to someone with cancer. The long-term effects of STIs include an impact on fertility, further complicating things for those who want to have children in the future. STIs such as chlamydia cause inflammation of the uterine tubes, preventing fertilization of the egg or leading to tubal pregnancy (where the fertilized egg grows outside of the uterus). Many women do not know when they have contracted an STI because they often have no symptoms, and yet damage is occurring internally. The best way to prevent STIs is by using male or female condoms all the time with everybody; this way you are also pre-venting unwanted pregnancy.

Websites

- **Fertile Hope** (www.fertilehope.org) is an initiative of the LIVESTRONG Foundation providing reproductive informa-tion, support, and hope to cancer survivors who are at risk for infertility.
- **The Oncofertility Consortium** (www.myoncofertility.org) is a national, interdisciplinary organization involved in the care of cancer survivors and their reproductive health.
- **SaveMyFertility.org** (www.savemyfertility.org), part of the En-docrine Society, is a resource for people with cancer who want to learn more about preserving their fertility before and during cancer treatment.
- **Fertile Future** (www.fertilefuture.ca) is a Canadian nonprofit organization that provides fertility preservation information and support services to people with cancer as well as oncolo-gy professionals.
- **The American Society for Reproductive Medicine** is the na-tionally and internationally recognized society for informa-tion, education, advocacy, and standards in the area of re-productive medicine. They have resources for patients (www .reproductivefacts.org) and professionals (www.asrm.org).

What Comes Next?

This chapter contains some hard facts to face, but there is also room for hope. We are learning more and more about fer-tility preservation, and what seems like a small chance for success today may be much better in just a few years. It is very important to talk about this with your partner, your parents if appropriate, and your healthcare team so that you can maximize your chances of protecting your ability to one day conceiving or creating a pregnancy.

References

Armuand, G.M., Rodriguez-Wallberg, K.A., Wettergren, L., Ahlgren, J., Enblad, G., Höglund, M., & Lampic, C. (2012). Sex differences in fertility-related information received by young adult cancer survivors. *Journal of Clinical Oncology, 30*, 2147–2153. doi:10.1200/JCO.2011.40.6470

Crawshaw, M.A., Glaser, A.W., Hale, J.P., & Sloper, P. (2009). Male and female experiences of having fertility matters raised alongside a cancer diagnosis during the teenage and young adult years. *European Journal of Cancer Care, 18*, 381–390. doi:10.1111/j.1365-2354.2008.01003.x

Gorman, J.R., Bailey, S., Pierce, J.P., & Su, H.I. (2012). How do you feel about fertility and parenthood? The voices of young female cancer survivors. *Journal of Cancer Survivorship, 6*, 200–209. doi:10.1007/s11764-011-0211-9

Niemasik, E.E., Letourneau, J., Dohan, D., Katz, A., Melisko, M., Rugo, H., & Rosen, H. (2012). Patient perceptions of reproductive health counseling at the time of cancer diagnosis: A qualitative study of female California cancer survivors. *Journal of Cancer Survivorship, 6*, 324–332. doi:10.1007/s11764-012-0227-9

Olatunbosun, O.A., & Zhu, L. (2012). The role of sperm banking in fertility preservation. *Clinical and Experimental Obstetrics and Gynecology, 39*, 283–287.

Peddie, V.L., Porter, M.A., Barbour, R., Culligan, D., MacDonald, G., King, D., … Bhattacharya, S. (2012). Factors affecting decision making about fertility preservation after cancer diagnosis: A qualitative study. *BJOG: An International Journal of Obstetrics and Gynaecology, 119*, 1049–1057. doi:10.1111/j.1471-0528.2012.03368.x

Salama, M., Winkler, K., Murach, K.F., Seeber, B., Ziehr, S.C., & Wildt, L. (2013). Female fertility loss and preservation: Threats and opportunities. *Annals of Oncology, 24*, 598–608. doi:10.1093/annonc/mds514

CHAPTER 6

Metastatic Disease and Palliative Care

S ometimes treatment fails, sometimes the cancer comes back in another organ, and sometimes the cancer has already spread beyond the primary site prior to diagnosis. This rightly qualifies as being unfair and just plain wrong. Recurrent or metastatic cancer often is treated with the aim of maintaining quality of life for as long as possible, until the end of life, rather than cure. Some people live with cancer as a chronic disease for years, but the prospect of end of life is still ever present. This is a difficult topic to think and read about. But, it is an important one that is often avoided precisely because it is uncomfortable.

The Cancer Has Spread—Now What?

Metastasis is a frightening reality for many with cancer, as well as their families and their healthcare providers. Despite great progress in cancer survival statistics, about 20% of people with cancer have disease that has spread to other parts of the body (Howlader et al., 2012). While some live with advanced cancer for years and in that time other treatments become available and life is extended, for others, there is not enough time and life is limited. It is especially difficult to think about for those who have not lived a long life. Thoughts of death often occur at the time of diagnosis, but these are not the same as when death is closer because of metastatic disease. Living with metastatic cancer is filled with uncertainty and, for some, a great deal of distress.

> *And then I get the news that it came back . . . it's redeveloping. I felt my world crashing around me again. I went from being very strong, like stone . . . and then I was broken into pebbles. I built myself back up. And now I was breaking down again. Knowing that I'm going to be losing my strength again, my pain tolerance, not being able to keep up with things . . .*
> —Daylan, B-cell leukemia

When life is limited, it is typical to think about the process of dying, which causes much anxiety for some. At or near the end of life, people are often concerned about pain. How much will it hurt? What if it can't be controlled? How will I cope? It is usual to grieve the loss of relationships that will occur after death. It is common to worry about how your family will cope financially and emotionally. As the cancer takes over the body, weakness and an inability to do the everyday things we take for granted—showering, making lunch, doing the laundry—rob us of the independence we want and expect.

The Five Stages of Grief

In the 1960s, a doctor by the name of Elisabeth Kübler-Ross suggested that there are five stages of grief: denial, anger, bargaining, depression, and acceptance. Her model became widely accepted in many different disciplines, though it also received criticism. But her book started a conversation about death and dying that had not happened before. Talking about death was a major taboo. This led to many people dying with a great deal of existential suffering; they had not been allowed to talk about it, even to their loved ones, and in turn their families had suffered their grief in silence (Kübler-Ross, 1969, 2005).

Denial: *"This is not happening to me."* This is usually a temporary stage and may be a defense against the sad reality of the situation. Denial can be conscious or unconscious and may allow the person to get things in order before accepting what lies ahead.

Anger: *"Why me? This is not fair!"* Once denial passes, some people react with anger—at themselves, the disease, God. Although the anger may not be rational, it is felt in a very real way.

Bargaining: *"If I can just have some more time, I'll trade . . . "* This stage represents the beginning of accepting the inevitable but with the hope that some reprieve is possible. The bargaining is often with some higher power and with the promise of leading a better life in exchange for more time.

Depression: *"My life is over; there's no use in even trying."* This stage is thought to represent the start of disengagement and withdrawal from loved ones. The sadness that this brings may be interpreted by others as depression.

Acceptance: *"I'm ready to die; it'll be okay."* This final stage is thought to represent an acceptance of the inevitability of death and, with it, an assumption that the anger and depression of earlier stages disappear. It is often assumed that this state of acceptance is in a way a state of grace, but this stage is widely criticized. Many people never come to terms with their own mortality or that of their loved ones and fight death to their very least breath.

This model has been misinterpreted by many. Here are some of the problems with it:

- It seems to suggest that you have to start at denial and work through all the stages.
- It does not mention the resilience and coping that many people show when dealing with grief.
- There is no set schedule or timeline.
- Some people don't experience any of these stages and yet still experience grief.
- It doesn't take culture into account. Different cultures have very different approaches to grief.
- It does not consider the family and how family members deal with grief in their own time and way.
- There is no mention of hope.

Advance Care Planning

Most young adults have not considered their own mortality and have certainly not made plans for what might happen at the end of their life. The American Academy of Pediatrics, the World Health Organization, and the Institute of Medicine suggest that young adults should play an active role, depending on their stage of development and desire to do so, in planning their care, including their wishes for end-of-life, or *palliative*, care. This can be challenging for parents and healthcare providers who think that talking about this takes away hope or suggests that they are giving up. Patients may be hesitant to talk about their wishes because they are fearful that by talking about end-of-life issues, they will be denied active treatment. And they also may be afraid of signaling to their family and friends that they are dying.

I'd tell them (someone with metastatic disease) just because they're metastatic, doesn't mean anything. It doesn't mean that they should stop fighting. It doesn't mean that they should think that their life is over because it's not. The only difference between them and the person beside them is that they know possibly what might kill them. But either one of them could always walk out their door and get hit by a bus the next day. With the therapies that are out there, there is so much hope for at least extended life. And you never know what happens in the future. You can live a long time with metastatic disease and it's worth it. It's worth having that life because who knows what comes after. You might as well enjoy what you have.

—Sarah, metastatic breast cancer

Young adults facing the end of life may feel disconnected from their peers with cancer who are in active treatment and seen as still "fighting" the disease. Avoiding talking to family, friends, and healthcare providers in an effort to protect them can be very isolating at a time when closeness and the ability to speak what is in your heart and mind are of utmost importance. Young people facing the end of life often feel that they have not accomplished their life goals and are not sure how they will be remembered. Healthcare providers or parents may question the competence of a young person in making end-of-life decisions even if the individual is of legal age. This is why an open discussion about end-of-life wishes should happen over time and not just in times of crisis or when death is near. Stating your wishes about treatment—including ending treatment—is important. It can give some control in a situation that feels uncontrollable and is one way of having some autonomy where choices are limited and in-dependence has largely been lost due to the illness.

It is suggested that advance care planning begin at the time of diagnosis and carry on throughout the disease process. This is not likely to happen if it is viewed as giving up or losing hope. The intent of advance care planning is to ensure that the voice and wishes of the patient are heard and complied with. Many studies have shown that this is important to young adults. One way of making your wishes known is to have an **advance health-care directive** (sometimes called a *living will*). The intent of this document is to let others know your wishes only if you can-not speak for yourself. It is not intended to replace your wish-es while you can still speak for yourself or communicate in any way. By indicating what you want, you can actually help your family, if the time comes when you cannot speak for yourself, by letting them know what you want so that they don't have to guess or argue with each other about your wishes.

Many examples of advance healthcare directives are avail-able, including one designed especially for young adults with cancer called "Voicing My Choices." It was developed by Ag-ing With Dignity, an organization that created a document for adults called Five Wishes®, and was tested in studies with young adults. You can use this document to appoint someone to speak for you if you are not able and also to list your choices regarding end-of-life care.

The document contains eight sections:

1. The person I want to make healthcare decisions for me when I can't make them for myself
2. My wish for the kind of medical treatment I want or don't want
3. My wish for how comfortable I want to be
4. My wish for how I want people to treat me
5. My wish for what I want my loved ones to know

6. Spiritual wishes
7. How I want to be remembered
8. My voice (blank pages for writing messages for people).

You can download this form from www.agingwithdignity .org/voicing-my-choices.php. It is suggested that you talk to your family and loved ones about what you have written or chosen from the checklist in the document so that they are aware of your wishes and can share their thoughts with you. It is also important that they know that this document exists and where to find it should you suddenly become ill. Your healthcare providers also need to know that you have completed it so they know your desires for care if you cannot speak for yourself.

Maximizing Quality of Life

Cancer care is a continuum from prevention to diagnosis and treatment, and then for some a transition from attempting to cure the disease to maintaining quality of life through to end-of-life care. For many, this is hard to even think about, but for others, end-of-life care is as important to plan for as was choosing treatment earlier on. When cure is no longer possible, the transition to palliative care is the next step. Some people think about palliative care as the same as terminal care, but that is not accurate. The objective of palliative care is to maximize quality of life through effective management of symptoms such as pain, shortness of breath, increasing weakness, and distress, both physical and emotional. Many cancer centers and hospitals today have palliative care teams that are available to help to reduce and manage distressing symptoms like pain and will support you to live the best way possible for as long as possible.

The 411 on Useful Websites
About Palliative and Hospice Care

- **Caring Connections** is the website (www.caringinfo.org) of the National Hospice and Palliative Care Organization. It has many useful resources, including how to find hospice care where you live.
- **The Center to Advance Palliative Care** website (www.getpalliativecare.org) has useful resources, such as links, a blog, videos, and tips on how to get palliative care and determine whether it is right for you.
- **The Canadian Virtual Hospice** (www.virtualhospice.ca) has a number of resources such as discussion forums, questions and answers, and a place to read and share personal stories. There are sections for you, your family and friends, as well as healthcare professionals.

Most adults prefer to die at home, and this may hold true for young adults, too. This may mean moving back in with your parents, which may work for some, but not for all. Hospice care can be provided in your home. You may need to pay for all or part of this care, with volunteers and family or friends providing the rest of your care. It is possible to rent a hospital bed to make it easier for your caregivers. You can also rent oxygen and other equipment to help when you are weak or unable to move with comfort. Inpatient hospice care is another choice—a home-like setting where care is provided by professional and support staff. This can be a little weird for young adults, as almost all the other residents are going to be much older.

Being Remembered

Every human being wants to be remembered by loved ones. For older people, their legacy may be two or more generations of children, grandchildren, and great-grandchildren. They may have created buildings or written books or taught generations of children, or found some other way to leave their mark on the world. But if you are just starting out in your career or have not yet had a family of your own, it can be difficult to see how you have made a difference. If you ask, your family and friends will no doubt share with you what you mean to them and how you have made their lives better, or more fun, or what you have taught them.

You can create a legacy in a number of ways. You can plant a tree or bulbs that will grow and flower and remind others of you for many years. You can make a video for each of your loved ones with special thoughts or memories. You can post videos on YouTube to reach a limitless audience. You can write letters to your family, including your young children, with your thoughts about them, the milestones they will reach without you, and how you would like to advise them even if you are not there in person. You can create a charitable foundation or support a cause so that others will benefit from your generosity for years to come. You can put together a time capsule (real or virtual) for your family and friends to open at certain times with items from your life with them or gifts that you want them to have in the future. You can spend time with loved ones now and create memories for all of you.

What Comes Next?

Even at the end of life, hope can exist. *Hope* has been described as a phenomenon that helps patients live life until the moment of death (Fanslow-Brunjes, 2008). Fanslow-Brunjes suggests that hope occurs across the complete cancer journey, from diagnosis where the hope is for cure, during treatment where the hope is for success, the constant hope for prolongation of life, and finally, hope for a peaceful death.

References

Fanslow-Brunjes, C. (2008). *Using the power of hope to cope with dying: The four stages of hope.* Sanger, CA: Quill Driver Books.

Howlader, N., Noone, A.M., Krapcho, M., Neyman, N., Aminou, R., Waldron, W., ... Cronin, K.A. (Eds.). (2012). SEER cancer statistics review, 1975–2009 (Vintage 2009 Populations) [Based on November 2011 SEER data submission, posted to the SEER website, April 2012]. Retrieved from http://seer.cancer.gov/csr/1975_2009_pops09

Kübler-Ross, E. (1969). *On death and dying.* New York, NY: Macmillan.

Kübler-Ross, E. (2005). *On grief and grieving: Finding the meaning of grief through the five stages of loss.* New York, NY: Scribner.

SECTION II. Being a Person

CHAPTER 7

Sexuality, Dating, and Relationships

I n emerging and young adulthood, people are more serious about forming permanent relationships and finding a potential life partner. So how do you manage to do this while coping with a new cancer diagnosis or getting through treatment, or dealing with the fallout from cancer long ago? For some people, this is not a problem, but for others, dating and being sexual pose significant challenges. Even if you have a partner, committed or not, body image issues and other physical changes can affect sexual desire and interest, as well as sexual response. In this chapter, you will read not only about what can happen but also about what you can do to help yourself and your partner(s) to overcome challenges to body image, sexuality, and relationships.

Is This "The One"?

What is dating like when you have or had cancer? Depending on the age when you had cancer, this can be difficult. You may have put dating and your social life on hold as you went through treatment. You may have missed out on many oppor-

tunities to interact with potential partners because you had to
avoid crowds when your blood counts were low, or you may
have spent months in the hospital before and after a bone marrow or stem cell transplantation. But your peers went on with
their lives, found partners, moved in together, got married,
started having children—and you got left behind.

> *Not having breasts definitely gives you issues when it
> comes to dating, because then you're like, "All right,
> how am I going to explain this?" And it's not like say-
> ing, "OK, not only do I not have breasts, but I also
> have cancer that I'm most likely going to die from at
> some point." Broaching that subject is not very easy.
> Not many guys say, "Oh sure, I want the cancer girl."
> A lot of guys my age would probably prefer taking a
> less complicated situation on. It doesn't help that I'd
> be a single mom and have a terminal illness and have
> no breasts. It's not really a selling point.*
>
> —*Sarah, metastatic breast cancer*

Quick Tips: How Do You Start Dating When You're Out of Practice or Out of the Loop?

- Don't take it too seriously. You're looking for company and some fun, not necessarily a soul mate or life partner.
- Practice asking someone to go out for coffee, a movie, or a walk (and yes, girls can do the asking too!).
- Say the words out loud to yourself in the mirror or to a friend.
- Think about what it means if someone says no. It's not the end of the world, and it doesn't mean you're not a great person. It just means that the person you asked is busy or not interested at the time, or perhaps already in a relationship.
- It gets easier with practice and time. Really.

Others find it really hard to date, or even think about dating, when they're dealing with cancer and treatment or afterward. Even though having someone to love and who loves and supports you is great, you may just not be able to make the effort to find and nurture a relationship. Or you may not have the energy to deal with problems in a relationship and let it continue way past its "sell-by" date. Sometimes it's easier to take the path of least resistance and just let things go on and on . . . whether alone or with someone who's not right. This book is not intended to tell you what to do—only you know what is right for you. There is no 100% right or wrong way to handle a situation or way to be. Just try to figure out why it's okay to live with the status quo, and if you decide that you can't, then do something to change it.

> *Had I not had cancer, I probably wouldn't have dated him, to be quite honest. I was very much like, "I'm not dating seriously right now," and, excuse my language, "but if you want to buy me dinner and have sex, sure, why not?" It went on for a couple months and two big "I'm not looking for anything serious" conversations until I was finally like, "That's it," and we ended up sleeping together after that, and then he turned out to be an asshole.*
> —Alison D., kidney cancer

One of the biggest issues that many people with cancer face is when to tell someone that they have or had cancer. When do you disclose, and how much? There is no perfect answer to this question. If you tell too early, you may scare the other person away. If you don't tell for an extended period of time, it may feel like you are hiding something important. Some people say that if you're dating someone, you should tell on the third or fourth date. Why then? Well, the first date is just too early. If you bring it up and then never see the person again, you may think that the cancer scared him or her off. This may be true, or the person may just not be interested in seeing you again for other reasons. But telling all on the first date may be too much, too soon.

The second date may also be too soon, but you may feel comfortable disclosing your history at this time. Just remember that some people might be scared off by your cancer history—and you wouldn't want someone like that in your life anyway because the cancer is part of who you are. So the third or fourth date is seen by many as the ideal time. You are not that invested in the other person yet, and hopefully the person is interested enough in you by this point that learning about the cancer is not too overwhelming.

I'm thankful that I married my husband and we have a solid relationship. I can understand it being pretty difficult for young women trying to meet a man. How do you approach that? I wouldn't do that on the first three dates. That's something that could wait until it's actually a little more serious and maybe if it comes up in conversation.

—Serena, non-Hodgkin lymphoma

Quick Tips: How Much Do You Tell?

- It all depends on what you are comfortable disclosing.
- A good place to start is to state simply "I had cancer ___ (months or years) ago."
- Wait for a response. If they don't say anything immediately, don't try to fill the silence. (This is big stuff, and they may need to collect their thoughts for a few moments.)

- If they change the subject, it may mean that they aren't able to process this and you need to ask them at another time what they think or feel about your disclosure.
- If they ask you to tell them more about what happened, you can start simply and allow their questions guide how much detail to give.

So, if you're ready to date again, how do you handle getting up close and personal with someone? First, you don't have to rush into anything. Having cancer may make you feel pressured to settle down and get intense pretty quickly. This can be off-putting for potential partners who may be in a very different place than you. On the other hand, you may feel as though you need to take more time before getting sexual with someone. You may be afraid to expose yourself physically or emotionally and need to get to know someone longer before sharing something private and intimate.

> It's difficult for me to think about dating anybody
> [else]. But it's even difficult to think about dating
> him right now. I feel like the kind of person I was as
> a sexual being has been stripped away. Small things,
> like not feeling comfortable in your own skin and in
> your own body and not feeling confident in the way
> you look. A lot of the side effects make me not want
> anyone to see me or judge me.
>
> —Naomi, Hodgkin lymphoma

Cancer survivors may want more serious relationships, or perhaps they hang on to relationships longer because they are afraid of never finding someone new to love and who will love them. For couples where one person is diagnosed with cancer, the end of the relationship is more likely due to the added stress that cancer brings, including financial problems, uncertainty, and sexual and fertility challenges (Kirchhoff, Yi, Wright, Warner, & Smith, 2012).

> *It's kind of sucky to go out and meet some guy and put him through everything that my husband had to go through that totally destroyed our marriage. To put that kind of stress on somebody else is asking a lot. So you can't really get mad when guys pretend to your face that they're OK with you saying that you have cancer but then don't call you ever again because it's kind of inevitable. But at least they're nice to your face. The cool thing is that you do get to go out once or twice. And you know when you go out with someone once or twice if they have a thing for you—if they found you attractive, if there was any sort of spark. And at least being able to go out and do that and feel that for a couple of days, that's better than nothing. At least you get that feeling where, "Yeah, I might be wearing strap-on boobs, but this guy is digging me." So you don't feel completely unfeminine anymore.*
>
> *—Sarah, metastatic breast cancer*

The Body, Altered

> *Before, my two favorite things about myself were my breasts and my hair. And those were the two things I lost with cancer. It's a horrible thing, breast cancer, because it takes those things away from you. And so it totally screws up your body image for a really long time. It's really hard to feel beautiful when you have*

no eyebrows, no hair. You have scars all over your frig-
gin' body.

— *Melinda, breast cancer*

Scars are an inevitable part of having cancer. In addition to the obvious surgical scars after mastectomy or abdominal surgery, other more subtle scars can affect your body image. If you've had chemotherapy, you'll likely have a scar on your chest or arm from the implanted IV line. This is often in a highly visible place and hard to hide. Many people gain a lot of weight quickly if they're on steroids such as dexamethasone, and they get stretch marks on their breasts, stomach, back, arms, and legs. These can be a constant reminder of the cancer. If you've had radiation, you might have small tattoos that were used for marking the treatment area. These are usually really tiny but also a reminder long after treatment is over. If the scar is visible even when wearing clothes, others may comment or ask about it. If the scar is usually hidden by clothing, going to the beach or pool may cause stares or questions. Getting naked in front of a new sexual partner may expose scars that are usually hidden from everyone but yourself.

I understand that surgeons are there to save your life.
But it wouldn't hurt to think of the cosmetics. Now
I have the scar on my chest, and it's fairly high up
near my collarbone. I notice people looking at it from
time to time. Most of the time it doesn't bother me. I'm
thinking in my head, "Oh, they must be looking at
my necklace." But then sometimes I get self-conscious
about it because I can feel it . . . and the nerves don't
feel right in that area.

— *Serena, non-Hodgkin lymphoma*

Scars change with time. What starts as something red and shiny will with time become pink, then silvery-white (or light brown, depending on your natural skin tone). If you develop a keloid scar (an overgrowth of skin that is raised and thick), ask your doctor or nurse for a referral to a plastic surgeon. The surgeon may be able to revise the scar or suggest treatment to improve what it looks like. You may experience altered sensations when the area of the scar is touched; numbness or a prickly feeling is common as the nerves regenerate. This can be unpleasant, even painful, or you may feel nothing at all. More about this later.

Quick Tips: Accepting Your Changed Body

- Spend some time in front of the mirror looking at your body.
- Think about what you like about your body instead of what is changed or different.
- Remind yourself that others will like those parts of you too.
- Ask a close friend to look at and describe your scars and your body; someone else's view may be quite different from your own.
- Talk to others with cancer and ask how they cope.
- We all have things that we don't like about our bodies—potential partners do, too.

It's really hard because I see myself in the mirror and I think, this isn't what I look like. This isn't what I used to look like. This is not me. But then I stop and think, "OK, well, six months ago, a year ago, I looked worse. And I had no hair. And I couldn't move my body. And I had this problem going on and that problem going on." So I have to stop myself and realize that even though I'm not where I necessarily want to be or think I should be, I'm here, and things are better than they used to be. But it's definitely hard. I have all the pictures of my husband and me, of what we used to be, pretransplant, prediagnosis. Sometimes I'll look at those pictures and get really upset. I think, I used to be so pretty, and I looked so happy, and all that kind of stuff. I have to just, unfortunately, live with what I have.

—Jennifer, acute myeloid leukemia

So how do you deal with stares and questions? One way is to use humor. Having a ready answer or comeback can be very helpful because you don't have to think about it; you can just use a well-practiced phrase without involving much thought or emotion. Something like, "Yeah, my mom told me never to get a tattoo from a drunk sailor" will discourage further questions.

Some survivors undergo plastic surgery to make a scar less noticeable. Others get a tattoo around and over the scar to make it a statement; a good offense can be better than any kind of defense. Some accept their scar as evidence of their experience and survival. Your friends can be really helpful—they can act as shields for you and protect you when others are nosy or mean. Some people try to hide scars as much as possible, even during sexual encounters. For example, you can wear a T-shirt to cover up a scar on your upper body at all times, including at the beach or the pool, or in sexual situations. Carefully placed scarves can hide scars on the lower body, or you can buy sexy underwear to hide scars on the lower part of your abdomen.

I said [to my husband], "Are you happy with this?" And he just looked at me. I said, "Can I please go ahead and do some tattooing?" And he says, "Yeah." So I came up with a design. I met with an artist and he agreed that he would tattoo over all my scars, ev-

ery single mastectomy scar, the port scar, the nipple scars. He made me this beautiful creation that I am very proud to show off now. Even with the deformity. So I have daisies for nipples. I have an ivy vine for my mastectomy scar, and I have the ribbon with my year of diagnosis with the word "hope" in it. That basically is what makes me a survivor.

—Aimee, breast cancer

It's sad that so many of us are ashamed of how we look, but since childhood, we have been told what looks all right and what doesn't. The media is a powerful influence in all of our lives, and most of us have grown up looking at images of "perfect" celebrities and athletes. What most of us ignore is that often those images are manipulated before being printed or put on the Internet. Also, many of those celebrities and athletes spend most of their day working really hard to look that way. The rest of us are studying or working full- or part-time jobs, not working out for six to eight hours a day.

I've a list of body issues so long that scars are way, way down at the bottom, and it's not really that big of an issue.

—Cheryl, cervical cancer

There is no right or wrong way to deal with physical imperfections. It's up to you to decide how you want to deal with it. We tend to judge ourselves much more harshly than others judge us. The fact is that when people are interested in you sexually, they are usually so turned on and motivated to be with you that they don't really see much at all. Healthy lust has a way of blurring the edges of our vision. Things like scars just aren't important in the moment. Of course, it's helpful to warn a sexual partner that you have a scar and how you feel about it—no one wants a surprise in the afterglow. Don't think that your sexual partner is 100% fine with the way he or she looks naked either!

> *I look at my wedding pictures and it makes me so upset because I married a wonderful man . . . and all I can see is that I had no breasts. . . . Everyone else sees nothing. But all I can see is that I was flat and I was wearing prosthetics.*
>
> *—Melinda, breast cancer*

What about missing parts? In some kinds of cancer, for example, sarcoma, amputation is necessary. You can't hide a missing arm or leg without clothes on, but you can do a pretty good job with a prosthesis and clothing. A missing breast (or two) can also be easily hidden, until it's time to be naked. In this situation, honesty and straightforwardness usually are best. Once again, give limited information to begin with, and wait. If people want more information, they'll ask for it. Getting used to a missing part is difficult. Some people get over it, while others continue to struggle with it.

> *That was one of my biggest selling points when I was in the dating world, I had really nice breasts. It was hard to change to not having that anymore. You kind of feel like a little boy when you don't have your clothes on. . . . To a guy, a pair of boobs is a pair of boobs. But when you're looking at a pair of mounds . . . because boobs aren't boobs without nipples, right? I did find that weird. It was one thing after the mastectomy and you just see this flat piece of skin with a scar where there used to be a real breast. But once it gets*

formed into the shape of a breast, it doesn't match the look of a breast . . .

—*Aimee, breast cancer*

Some people gain weight because of the treatments they have, or they lose weight or muscle mass. Hair loss is common with chemotherapy, and sometimes your hair just never grows back the same way. It's not uncommon for cancer survivors to have very a negative outlook on how attractive they are. This can affect your self-confidence, and so you may never try to date or think that no one will ever want to date you.

For those with a partner, it can still be scary to expose your naked self. Your partner's reaction may be very influential in how you see yourself. Some people hide from their partner's view and dress and undress in the bathroom or closet. While this may protect your feelings, it deprives your partner of an important sensual experience. Our partners like to see us naked—and we like to see them naked, too! Our partners see past the imperfections that we tend to focus on and get turned on by the things that they see. Most people, when asked, say that they love the essence of their partner, not individual body parts. Think about that for a moment: Why do you love your partner? Is it because of a washboard stomach or dimples, or because he or she is kind and funny and has been supportive through your cancer experience? Your partner loves you because you are smart and funny and have been brave and resourceful in the face of cancer.

You shouldn't need someone else to tell you that you're beautiful, but that's what helped me, having my husband there reassuring me. He was there basically telling me that I was sexy the entire time.

—*Melinda, breast cancer*

Quick Tips: How to Adapt to Your New Body

- Accept that it can take a year or even more to get used to the new you.
- Try to wear your pre-cancer clothes. Dressing the way you used to can help make you feel like you used to and will help you cope with the changes.
- Makeup can help you feel better, but you have to take the effort to use it.
- Working out, or just getting some form of activity, can help you feel better about your body. (Exercise helps in many other ways, too, which will be discussed in the next chapter.)
- If you just can't move on and accept your new self, think about getting support.
- A friend or family member may be able to provide you with the support you need. Or, you may need to see a professional who can help.
- Ask your nurse or doctor to refer you to a social worker or a sexuality counselor or therapist.

> *To me, the most important thing was the reconstruction. Do research about it and don't accept what a plastic surgeon tells you until you look around and see. They may be telling the truth, but look around, ask questions, do research, and look online. It's important to get that outcome that you want because it's going to be for the rest of your life.*
>
> —*Melinda, breast cancer*

Talking About It

Sexuality is a broad concept that covers who you think you are as a sexual person, whom you are attracted to, what your dreams and fantasies are, whom you choose to be sexual with, and what you do sexually. It is often confused with intimacy, or the word *intimacy* is used instead of *sex* or *sexual activity*. Intimacy really means that heart-to-heart connectedness that we may have with one or more people in our lives. It's really good if your sexual partner is also your intimate partner, but it's possible to not have sex with someone you are very intimate (close) to, and to not feel close (intimate) with a sexual partner.

Cancer treatments affect sexuality, but it's often not talked about by cancer doctors and nurses. That's a BIG problem because you need to know what might happen so that you can be prepared. Because healthcare providers are usually silent about this, getting help can be a bit of a challenge. Most oncology care providers say that they are prepared to answer questions from patients—they just want the patient to ask the question first. You may wonder why no one from your healthcare team has brought up the topic or asked you if you're doing all right in this area. That's not unusual; doctors and nurses don't ask about it because they're embarrassed, they've had little education about it, they think that your sex life is none of their business, or they don't have a lot of time to talk to you about it. This is a great pity, because 80% of all cancer survivors have some problems with sexuality, but they are asked about it less than 20% of the time! In one study of young adult survivors of childhood cancer, 43% of those asked said that they had at least one problem related to sexuality. Young women had more problems than young men (Zebrack, Foley, Wittmann, & Leonard, 2010). The study also found that sexual problems were associated with less overall life satisfaction.

Having the "sex talk" with healthcare providers can be even more challenging if you're gay, lesbian, bisexual, or transgender (GLBT). You may have encountered some homophobia or heterosexism from healthcare providers (hopefully not) or in other situations and may be too tired, scared, or depressed to deal with explaining who you are and what you do (even though you shouldn't have to). Society has to change, and many would suggest that it *is* changing, although perhaps not as fast as we may like. Your healthcare providers need to take care of YOU, the whole you, not just the organ(s) affected by the cancer. They need to know if you are GLBT (they may know this from your records if you've had hormones or surgery) because that is a very important part of who you are as a person and those whom you love and share your life with, which is important in your overall plan of care. Most healthcare providers will say that they don't really care whom you choose to love or be sexual with and that they treat everyone the same. However, if you are GLBT-identified, you may have had past experiences with the healthcare system that have been hurtful or harmful.

It can be difficult to talk about sexuality or sexual difficulties with healthcare providers who are older than you (or look like they might faint at the thought of talking about it). But, they are more resilient than you may think, and they are also sexual beings under the white coats. The best thing to do is to just be matter-of-fact about what you need to tell them. Don't worry about what they're thinking or feeling. Most of the time, they're just glad that you asked the question because they couldn't figure out how to raise the topic. Start simple and see where the discussion goes. If they are really uncomfortable or don't answer your questions or take you seriously, find someone else to ask. Most survivors have a "go-to" person on their team—a favorite nurse or social worker or psychologist whom they can talk to and who will know where to make a referral if the problem needs more than talking to sort out.

The 411 on Having "The Talk" With Your Oncology Care Provider

Say what you mean. No beating around the bush!
- "When my partner touches my _____, it feels numb. Why is that?"
- "The last time I masturbated I noticed that _____. What can be done about this?"
- "How will I know when it's OK to have oral sex/go down on someone?"
- "What precautions does my partner need to know about if we want to _____?"
- And don't worry if you blush; it can't be controlled. And if your oncology care provider blushes, the same applies.

S-E-X: More Than a Three-Letter Word

What about sex? Sex is great—let's get that out of the way. But so is a good meal, a great book, or an iced tea or coffee (or cold beer) on a hot Saturday afternoon. Sex gets a lot of attention in the media, on blogs, and in books. We spend a lot of time talking about it, thinking about it, wanting it, and avoiding it . . . but not a lot of time learning about it.

> *Although important, sex isn't anything that my husband and I base our marriage on, which also makes me realize how much he really loves me. Although, like I said, it is important; it's a factor.*
> —*Aimee, breast cancer*

Cancer can and does change things sexually for many people. To be more accurate, it's the treatment of the cancer that causes most of the problems. Earlier in this chapter we talked about body image and how scars, missing parts, and an altered body can affect your self-image. But cancer treatment can also cause other changes that make sex more difficult, including anatomic and physiologic changes.

The sex life just diminished for multiple reasons. We didn't have the ability to . . . because I was in the hospital the entire time. And, you don't have the strength. You don't have the desire. You don't feel that great. You sure as hell don't feel sexy at all.

—*Jennifer, acute myeloid leukemia*

Guy Stuff

Let's start with what changes are possible for men. Surgery or radiation treatment to the pelvis may directly affect sex organs. The prostate is found deep in the pelvis, below the bladder. The function of the prostate is to provide fluid that mixes with sperm from the testicles (this is called *ejaculate*), and this then leaves the body through the penis during orgasm. On the outside of the prostate are the nerves that cause erections; any damage to these nerves during surgery or radiation can affect how they work and cause problems either in having or keeping an erection. For someone with colorectal cancer, a combination of surgery, radiation, and chemotherapy is usually the recommended treatment. The sexual side effects that may result include erectile problems and perhaps alterations with orgasm or ejaculation. In men, chemotherapy can cause damage to the testicles so that they don't produce sperm or enough testosterone.

Surgical removal of one or both testicles because of testicular cancer affects body image (although a prosthesis, an egg-shaped "false" testicle, is usually offered to replace the one removed). It also may reduce the amount of testosterone produced and may affect future fertility, as discussed in Chapter 5.

> *[I had] lots of issues around my illness and how I*
> *managed it and how it affected her. In retrospect, I*
> *think she got very irritated that I was feeling this way.*
> *I wasn't feeling very sexually driven or anything.*
> *And she was irritated because I wasn't making that*
> *more an issue with my doctors.*
>
> —*Stuart, acute lymphoblastic leukemia*

Girl Stuff

Surgery or radiation to the pelvis in women can also affect things sexually. Removing the ovaries will cause an immediate loss of hormones that affect sexual desire and arousal. Removing the uterus can change how orgasm is experienced. It also takes away your periods and your ability to become pregnant and have a baby, which may influence your feelings of femininity. Surgery to remove the cervix or radiation treatments to the cervix can make the vagina shorter and tighter and can make penetration painful.

> *I felt like my sex drive disappeared. There's so much*
> *else on my mind and so much stress, and I find myself*
> *going days and weeks without even really thinking*
> *about it. But I do miss the intimacy and the emotion-*
> *al aspect of being in a relationship, and the comfort*
> *of knowing somebody loves you and is supporting and*
> *caring for you.*
>
> —*Naomi, Hodgkin lymphoma*

Removal of one or both breasts not only affects body image but also sexual response. Many women say that their breasts are a very important trigger for their sexual response. Although having reconstruction will fix how you look, reconstructed breasts often do not react the same way that your own breasts do or did, and this can be a big loss for women. Some rare cancers (of the vagina or vulva) are treated with extensive surgery that takes away sexual feeling and even the ability to have intercourse.

> *It's very challenging to live your life to the fullest when you always have it haunting you, especially when you're dealing with the cosmetic effects of what it does. For women who have the estrogen component, that adds into it as well because you're always reminded of, "Oh my gosh, my mood swings or my hot flashes or my sex drive . . . My husband's upset with me because I'm not having sex and I don't care about my husband because I can't even care about myself right now." So I think it makes it very difficult for women to live their life fully. You try your best.*
>
> —*Kim, metastatic breast cancer*

For those with cancer affecting the brain, the radiation you had often interferes with the sex hormones your body produces. This happens because a part of your brain (the hypothalamus and pituitary gland) is exposed to radiation, which interrupts the signals to produce sex hormones. If your own sex hormones aren't enough and you experience problems, your doctors may give you hormone supplementation to normalize the levels.

Chemotherapy can cause the same kind of damage to the production of sex hormones. Chemotherapy can shut down a woman's ovaries, and after that, she may not produce enough estrogen. Sex hormones affect different aspects of healthy sexual functioning (for example, getting turned on) as well.

Do Something About It!

I'm only 30 and I'm married and my husband is only 31. I have low sex drive because of menopause and some of the medications I'm on. So we have to deal with that. And we work at that a lot because we have a long marriage ahead of us. That's something that my online support group talks about a lot because there's not much that doctors really talk to us about. So it's really frustrating. I know a lot of people that I've talked to are embarrassed to talk about it, and I'm not. So I find it frustrating that there are a lot of people who just don't do anything about it. I know their marriages suffer, and I find it really sad. But I always tell people that if it's a huge problem for you, you need a different oncologist because you're going to be married. If you're married and you're having sex, you need to do something about it.

—Melinda, breast cancer

So what can you do about these sexual problems? For men, different treatments are available to help you have an erection.

First, there are the pills: the class of drugs called *PDE-5 inhibitors*. These include Viagra® (sildenafil), Cialis® (tadalafil), and Levitra® (vardenafil) and a new pill called Stendra™ (avanafil). They work by preventing blood from leaving the penis once you get it in there by manual stimulation. They do NOT cause erections. In someone who has a real medical reason for taking them (not just for fun), they are unlikely to cause an erection lasting more than four hours as the ads on TV suggest. They are the easiest way to treat erectile problems, but they are expensive and often health insurance won't pay for them.

New formulations are becoming available, including a pill or film that you put under your tongue (this is another form of Levitra). A number of new medications are still in the clinical trial phase of development. All of these medications have side effects (mostly headache, nasal stuffiness, facial flushing, backache, and heartburn) and are not recommended for anyone who has very low blood pressure or is on treatment for chest pain. These pills are only available with a prescription from your doctor or nurse practitioner. You should never buy them online or from a friend or stranger, as they may be fake and contain ingredients (like rabbit poop—no kidding!) that can hurt you.

If the pills don't work, and if you don't have erectile nerves after surgery they probably won't, there are other things you can try. Penile pumps draw blood into the penis mechanically, and the blood is then kept in the penis by a tight rubber band at the base of the penis. Some men like this method, whereas others find it painful. The rubber band can only stay on for 30 minutes, and the penis feels cold because of the lack of blood flow while the rubber band is on. You can buy these pumps at sex stores and online. Or you can get a "medical device" with a prescription, but these are usually very expensive.

Another method that is very effective is the penile injection into the side of the penis. It may sound scary, but the needle is very small. This method really works, even for guys who don't have erectile nerves. Some porn actors use this method to stay hard for long periods of time, although that is not recommended as they are usually using too much and this causes something called *priapism*—an erection that just won't quit. While that might sound like fun, it hurts (a lot) and damages the penis. Do not try this at home! You need a prescription from your doctor for this medication.

And what's out there for women? Unfortunately, not a whole lot. There are no pills for loss of sexual interest, the most common complaint for women. There are things you can do for vaginal and vulval dryness, however. The best way to treat dryness is to figure out the cause and then treat it. Estrogen is the hormone of arousal, so if your ovaries were removed, you will have less estrogen (some is still produced in your body fat). If your cancer is not hormone dependent, then you should be getting estrogen replacement and you can use estrogen cream or pills in the vagina or on the vulva to keep things moist and comfortable. If your cancer is hormone dependent, then you may not be able to use any kind of estrogen replacement. It's important to talk to your cancer care providers about this. Some think that a little local estrogen cream on the dry tissues is OK because there is very little absorption and circulation to the rest of the body, while others won't allow this at all.

If you don't want to use estrogen, you can use a vaginal moisturizer like Replens®. This will help you feel more comfortable during the day but is not good for sexual activity. (More about that in the next section.) You can also use vitamin E oil (prick the capsule) on the tissues of the vulva and vagina. It is cheap and effective. These moisturizers don't solve the problem; they are a temporary fix. But they do not cause any harm and do not contain hormones.

Do NOT use any other kind of oils. Some people think that "natural" oils like olive oil or coconut oil are safer. However, they may contain pesticides and herbicides and can stay in the vagina, and with your body heat, they may turn rancid.

For any kind of sexual activity—with a partner or alone—using a good lubricant will make things much more comfortable and a whole lot of fun. There are some things you should know when buying and using a lube.

Lube 101: The Rules for Buying and Using a Lubricant

- K-Y® Jelly (the stuff in the doctor's office) is a BAD lube. It gets sticky quickly.
- The simpler the better. The fewer ingredients listed on the box, the better the product usually is.
- Avoid lubes that are "warming," "cooling," or "intensifying." They contain irritants and can burn delicate tissue.
- Watch out for perfumes and flavors for the same reason.
- Water-based lube can be reactivated with water if it dries out and is easy to wash off.
- Silicone-based lube (the ingredients list will have words ending with "-cone") can only be removed with soap and water.
- Don't use silicone lube with silicone sex toys—it destroys them!
- Go to a reliable sex store for help, and don't let them up-sell you. You can also get great lubes at your local drugstore (near the condoms) or online.

While a lot of what you've just read is about intercourse and penetration, remember that you can have a really great time, and relationship, without this. Most women have an orgasm with clitoral stimulation much easier than with penetration, and the same goes for oral sex. Guys get off with manual or oral stimulation too. Sexual activity should be like a buffet: many dishes, some hot, some cold, to try and taste. Limiting your sex life to just penetration is like only eating the salad from the buffet and ignoring the rolls, the cheese, and the dessert!

The Nasty Bits

I have bloating and a lot of bowel discomfort, so my stomach feels icky, and the idea of somebody touching it or holding it is really kind of disgusting to me right now. Also, with hair loss, I don't feel really very feminine or pretty, and I can't shave or wax because of the risks of nicking myself and getting an infection, or getting ingrown hairs and then those getting infected. All the normal hygienic routines you would do to make yourself feel pretty, I can't really do.

—Naomi, Hodgkin lymphoma

Some of the least talked about topics are how cancer and its treatments can mess up your body and your sex life. There are things that can happen that no one (except another cancer survivor) will talk to you about. While we can't cover everything that might affect your sex life, here are some common problems and solutions.

Constipation: Pain medications such as opioids can make you really constipated. That can lead to bloating, and for women, real discomfort if you insert anything into the vagina (dildo, finger, penis) because the rectum lies right behind the vagina. Stool softeners can help, or your doctor or nurse practitioner can prescribe a gentle laxative. But it's best to try to avoid getting constipated in the first place. Drink lots of water and eat fresh fruits and vegetables and whole-grain, high-fiber foods. If all else fails, the occasional use of a gentle enema before sex may be the only solution. Check with your healthcare provider first and get one from the drugstore.

Anal fissures: Related to constipation, straining to produce stool (or poo, for those of you who don't like medical terms) can cause tears in the skin around the anus. This hurts (a lot), especially if anal play or penetration is part of your sexual repertoire. You really do have to talk to your healthcare provider about this because they can take a long time to heal, and infection is always a possibility. Don't force anything in or out if you have pain or bleeding in that area. And tell your health-care provider if you have bleeding—it is never normal to bleed from there.

Vaginal/vulval sores: Many different kinds of chemothera-py cause mouth sores. The mouth is lined with mucous mem-branes. The vulva and vagina are too, so you can get the same kind of sores "down there" as you do in your mouth. If this happens, (a) tell your healthcare providers, and (b) practice very careful hygiene. That means washing gently with water only or a mild soap (Dove® for sensitive skin) or a cleans-er that does not have soap in it (like Cetaphil®) and patting dry very gently with a clean cotton towel afterward. Rinse with water after passing urine. Don't wear tight underwear or clothes, and try to go "commando" (no underwear) for as long as you can, especially when you nap or sleep. Don't have any kind of vaginal penetration, including use of a tampon, vibrator, or dildo.

Post-traumatic stress syndrome (PTSS) symptoms: Some people have long-lasting and powerful responses to treat-ment, procedures, and examinations (see Chapter 3). Being sexual can trigger flashbacks and cause you to panic, freeze, or completely freak out. It helps if you're in a safe and com-mitted relationship where your partner can support you as you explore your feelings about being sexual again and what, if any, response you have. It can be a little scarier if you don't have a regular partner and are sexual with someone you don't know well. If you are having symptoms of PTSS, you should be seeing a psychologist or social worker. You should talk to them about this and ask about what you can do if you're in bed with someone and start to feel panicked or scared. If you haven't been diagnosed with PTSS and you have uncon-trolled feelings when you're with someone sexually, you need to get help for this.

It's All About the Brain

There are two very important aspects of being sexually healthy that we have not talked about yet: communication and self-discovery. Let's start with communication.

> *I decided that when I met him I was going to be really honest and really open and just put it on the table right away. I told him on the first date. I didn't want to dance around the subject. I just let him know and then I just kind of explained it to him, and I said, "Do you have questions? I'm an open book; talk to me about it." And I've been really open from the beginning about my cancer diagnosis so I think that has helped me. I think it's better for people to know than to wonder and to have questions and make assumptions. And he said, "I can tell that this is something that you're uncomfortable with and you need to realize that it's not an issue for me. Everybody has things about their body that they're insecure about. You know I have my own as well. And this isn't something that should be affecting you. You need not to be so emotional about it; it's not a big deal." And it floored me because I'm thinking, "It is a big deal here. Man, you should care." But he doesn't. And most women that I know that have been through this, their husbands don't care either. But it's hard as a woman to recognize that and to accept that.*
>
> *—Allison, breast cancer*

The brain is the biggest sex organ in the body (really). Your imagination is contained in the brain. The brain also controls your thoughts and your words. You need to be able to talk to a sexual partner about what you want. We are not whales and dolphins—squeaks and grunts just don't cut it if you want to tell your partner what feels good and what you'd rather avoid. You need to be able to use words to tell him or her that you don't feel like sex because you're tired, not in the mood, distracted, doing the laundry, etc. This way your partner won't get the wrong idea and think that he or she is not attractive, has bad breath, or is a bad lover. It can be hard to talk about something that is so private and that you may never have talked about before. But this is the only way that your partner will know what you really want and like. It's sometimes difficult to talk about, mostly because many of our role models (such as our parents and teachers) didn't talk about sex openly.

> *I met a good man, is how I did it. It's all I can say. It was scary. It's not an easy thing to do. And man, I don't envy those [single] women. I feel for them because I know how hard it is to broach that subject, much less be intimate with somebody. Even if they know that you've had the surgery, it's still a whole new level to let them actually physically see you. For me it was, anyways.*
>
> *—Allison, breast cancer*

Quick Tips: Talking About Sex and Relationships

- Don't make assumptions about what your partner is thinking or feeling.
- Talk in "I" statements and allow your partner talk for and about himself or herself.
- Don't talk about sexual problems in bed or while naked.
- Listen (*really listen*) to what your partner has to say.

- Validate (I hear what you're saying) instead of fighting (no, I don't!).
- Think about writing down what you want to say in a letter.
- Schedule time to talk about what you've written.
- Some couples need help talking about sensitive topics. Consider seeing a therapist or counselor.

Bad and Sad Endings

I never really felt the kind of support that I thought could have been there, but I felt a lot of narrative around it, such as, "I'm losing my identity to your cancer." She talked a lot about how it really bothered her that everybody, when they talked to her, would ask her, "How's Stu doing?" That was the first thing they'd ask her, because I heard that all the time. And I get that. But (a) there's nothing I can do about it, and (b) it's not that unreasonable to expect that people would ask that question the most. So, yeah, there were probably coping issues for me, and from her end, too.

—Stuart, acute lymphoblastic leukeima

Not all relationships survive the cancer experience. Some couples just can't figure out how to support each other, and despite loving each other, the relationship ends. Unrelated issues often complicate things: children, money, family, fear, doubt, insecurity, and jealousy, and not everyone acts honorably, kindly, and lovingly. It's sad, but if you aren't getting what you need or want, you may have to separate for a while (or forever) in order to take the best care of yourself that you can. And ditto for your partner. There will be guilt, hurt feelings, complications, and anger. But if cancer teaches you nothing else, it is that life is short and nothing is certain. You have a right to be safe and happy and be loved, treasured, and cared for.

> *The cancer definitely complicated things. The stress and the financial aspects of the cancer—it all adds up after a while. We had our issues, like every couple has, anyway. But the cancer definitely didn't help. There were a lot of other underlying issues that we were dealing with. And I think the biggest problem with the cancer is that once you have cancer, the communication lines get blurred. And if you don't communicate enough, you know, your relationship just falls apart. I think because I was the patient, he stopped communicating with me because he thought I was dealing with enough already. But he wasn't getting enough help in dealing with his side of things because it affected him as well. Asking for help and making sure that you're taking care of yourself, even though you're taking care of somebody else, and being able to communicate with one another—we just lost that. There are intimacy issues as well, because I went into menopause. Well, we're not really 100% sure, but pretty sure, that I'm going through menopause.*
>
> *—Sarah, metastatic breast cancer*

Going Solo

In order to know what you really want and like, YOU have to know what your body can do. And there's really only one good way to learn about this: self-discovery. By that I mean more than masturbation. I mean you need to know how every part of your body looks and feels and reacts. This is easier for guys whose sexual parts are highly visible. For women, some mirror time is necessary to really look at all the parts of you, and to touch and feel and know what feels good and what feels great and what you want your partner (now or one day in the future) to touch and explore. Masturbation is great, too. It relieves tension, can help distract you from pain (physical and emotional), makes you feel good, helps you to get to sleep, and probably could end war if enough people did it instead of fighting! It also teaches you how your body reacts and what it feels like, and you can then show your partner what you like.

While some people are real experts at self-pleasuring (aka, masturbation), others need some help. The best thing that you can do to enhance your solo experience (and it's great for couples and both sexes) is to get a vibrator. These come in many shapes and forms, different price levels, and one (or five!) may not be enough. Men and women can use them, internally or externally. Just make sure that you are using the appropriate toy for the appropriate body part.

There are many places to get sex toys: online, in sex stores, and in drugstores (a regular wand massager for backs and necks is great for clitoral or penile/testicular stimulation). The following are some reputable suppliers where you can browse and buy. One of the advantages of actually going into a store is that you can see, feel, and play with the various toys that they sell.

- Adam and Eve: www.adameve.com
- Blowfish: www.blowfish.com
- Come as You Are (in Canada): www.comeasyouare.com
- Eve's Garden: www.evesgarden.com
- Good Vibrations: www.goodvibes.com
- Pure Romance: www.pureromance.com
- Babeland: www.babeland.com

What Comes Next?

This chapter has been about body image, dating, and sex, three important aspects of life and quality of life. You may have read some things you didn't think you needed to know about and some suggestions that may have helped. Sex is a basic human need, like food, water, and sleep, but it is so much more (and at times, so much less). And it needs a body that is well taken care of. So turn the page; the next chapter will talk about nutrition and exercise.

References

Kirchhoff, A.C., Yi, J., Wright, J., Warner, E.L., & Smith, K.R. (2012). Marriage and divorce among young adult cancer survivors. *Journal of Cancer Survivorship, 6,* 441–450. doi:10.1007/s11764-012-0238-6

Zebrack, B.J., Foley, S., Wittmann, D., & Leonard, M. (2010). Sexual functioning in young adult survivors of childhood cancer. *Psycho-Oncology, 19,* 814–822. doi:10.1002/pon.1641

CHAPTER 8

Nutrition, Exercise, and Supplements

This chapter could be summed up in just a few words: eat well and exercise, and if you do that, don't worry about supplements. That's it, nothing more and nothing less. But I have to say more than just those few words, so please continue reading! An overwhelming amount of evidence shows that eating well and exercising regularly is not only good for everyone, but for those with a history of cancer, it's essential. Why? Let's start with eating well and the components of a nutritious diet.

Eating Well

One of the biggest things for me is food because I love to cook. I'm a foodie. I love experiencing food and cooking it as well. So that was one of the choices I lost. Actually I couldn't eat lots of seafood. I couldn't eat sushi. Love sushi. I couldn't eat certain things and I was encouraged to cook my own food, which was fine for me and that wasn't too much of a difficulty. But food was the first thing that was removed from me.

—Jomar, acute lymphoblastic leukemia

Maintaining a healthy weight is important both during and after treatment. During treatment you may lose weight if you are unable to eat because of nausea, vomiting, altered taste, mouth sores, fatigue, and just feeling sick. If you were skinny going into treatment, you have to be extra careful to not lose more weight because this can affect your body's ability to heal from surgery, radiation, and chemotherapy. If you were overweight when starting treatment, you may lose weight because of not feeling well or any of the side effects of treatment mentioned previously. But the weight loss may also put you at risk for complications if you lose muscle mass in addition to fat. Some treatments for cancer cause weight gain, so if you were overweight to begin with, you may struggle with clothes that don't fit, joint pain, getting short of breath with physical activity, and not feeling good about what you see in the mirror.

I've always been a skinnier guy. And to finally be filled out and big and fill out shirts, it was great to me. And I loved food, and I just couldn't get enough food. But once that party was over, [I] lost the weight and now I have a bunch of stretch marks all over my body, but that's a small price to pay.

—Brian, leukemia

Nutritional Aims While in Treatment

- Achieve or maintain a healthy weight for you.
- Preserve muscle mass.
- Minimize side effects related to nutrition.
- Maximize quality of life.

So how do you do this? If you are *underweight or at risk of being underweight*, eat smaller meals more often and make them count. Eat foods that are dense in calories, which usually are foods that contain fat. Yay, ice cream! Don't worry about the warnings that fat is not good for you; this is the best way to get lots of calories with minimum effort. This works if you find that you get full really quickly when trying to eat normal-sized portions. Don't drink with your meals, including water and juice, because this makes you feel full faster. Drink between meals to keep hydrated.

If your weight is normal, you should have a balanced diet as suggested by the U.S. Department of Agriculture (see www .choosemyplate.gov) and Health Canada (www.hc-sc.gc.ca/ fn-an/food-guide-aliment/index-eng.php). A balanced diet is made up of

- **Fruits and vegetables:** the brighter the color, the better for you. Eat 10 servings a day (one serving = ½ a cup, so an apple is two servings). Whole fruit is better than juice.
- **Whole grains and legumes:** brown rice, beans, pasta, etc. Check the label to make sure that "whole grains" is listed first or second. Eat three servings a day (one slice of whole grain bread = 1 serving; ½ cup of brown rice = 1 serving)
- **Protein:** eggs, fish, meat, and chicken. Eat just one cup a day (about the size of a pack of cards). Dairy (cheese, yogurt, milk) counts as a protein but is high in fat and should be eaten in moderation.

What if you're a *vegetarian?* If you eat eggs and dairy products, you can quite easily maintain a healthy diet. You probably know how to make the most out of vegetable proteins such as beans, nuts and nut butters, peas, and soy products (use with caution if you're a woman and have an estrogen-dependent cancer). Eat whole-grain carbohydrates (brown rice, pasta, and whole-grain breads) and lots of fruit and vegetables.

Vegans need to make sure they eat enough plant-based pro-teins (nuts, legumes, and whole grain products) to ensure they are getting enough vitamin B_{12}. If not, they may need to take supplements. In the United States, vitamin D is added to most dairy products, but vegans may need to take supplements if

they don't get enough sun exposure (such as in the winter and in north-ern climates), which pro-vides the body with a sup-ply of vitamin D.

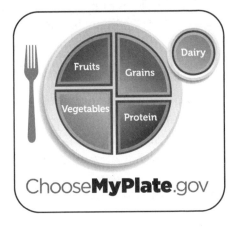

This is how the U.S. Department of Agricul-ture suggests that you divide the various com-ponents of every meal. Fruits and vegetables (cooked or raw) should make up half the plate. The rest should be grains and protein, with more grains than protein, and last-ly, a small amount of dairy products.

> *Everything that's organic is more expensive. The healthy stuff's always more expensive. But we have a great farmers' market in the summertime. And I try to grow my own vegetables in my backyard in the sum-mertime. But living in New England, in the winter-time, I have to survive off of what's at the grocery store for produce.*
> —*Sarah, metastatic breast cancer*

Should you try to eat only organic food? Food that is la-beled *organic* is controlled by the U.S. Department of Agricul-ture and is free from pesticides, hormones, and antibiotics.

There is no evidence to support that organic food will prevent cancer or a recurrence, and organic food has not been shown to be better nutritionally than regular food. This may not make sense to us, but that is what the studies show. It does tend to be more expensive, and you should never cut down your overall intake to save money to buy organic food. Organic food also tends to spoil more quickly, so you have to buy smaller quantities or risk having to throw away more. Pesticides are found on the outside of fruits and vegetables, so washing produce well and peeling fruits and vegetables before eating can help to avoid exposure to pesticides if you don't have access to organic produce.

> *I'm a single mom on a really strict budget, so I do the best that I can. Not all of us can afford to buy expensive juicers and go crazy. When you first get diagnosed, everybody and their brother sends you books on what you should and shouldn't be eating. I'm not living off of asparagus only or just pomegranates or anything. But I do the best that I can for being a single mom with an 11 year-old son that wants to eat everything and on a low income.*
>
> —*Sarah, metastatic breast cancer*

Going to a farmers' market is a really great way of learning about fruits, vegetables, and whole grains while supporting the local economy. Sometimes it is also cheaper than buying at your local supermarket. But what you find at the farmers' market may not be organic. Many farmers use pesticides, so you have to ask. It's great to talk to the farmers and learn about what they love to do, and you may be tempted to try vegetables and fruits that you've never eaten before. Often the produce you buy at the farmers' market is much dirtier than what you buy in the supermarket. Make sure to wash it well and to wash your hands prior to eating.

Juicing is another way that people try to consume their daily requirements of fruits and vegetables. Because all fiber is removed in the process, you don't get the benefits of that, but it can be a way to consume vegetables that you don't love (spinach, perhaps?) by combining them with flavors that you do like (berries or bananas are often used to hide the taste of vegetables). Juices tend to be less filling than whole fruit and do contribute calories to your diet, so if you want to control your calories, think twice about what fruits you're adding to your juicer.

There's been a lot written about *sugar* and how it can "feed" cancer. There is no evidence that eating foods with added sugar has any impact on the cancer itself. However, sugar is an "empty" calorie that doesn't add nutritional value to your diet. Soda, candy, and other high-sugar foods also interfere with your appetite so you are less likely to eat nutritious food. And they cause blood sugar levels to rise quickly and then drop, leaving you hungry, irritable, and tired. Of course, you don't have to avoid candy, chocolate, or sodas forever. Just try to make them treats and not part of your everyday consumption.

> *I shouldn't say I've changed my eating habits drastically because I've always eaten pretty healthily, but I try to eat a lot more whole foods and home-cooked meals. I don't eat out very much. And I have to watch what I eat because of bowel problems. Lots of prunes. "How can I add prunes to this meal? How can I mash prunes into this chili?" And then the rest of the family wonders why they keep having to go to the bathroom. My little secret.*
>
> *—Naomi, Hodgkin lymphoma*

Is there a better way to cook food? Steaming and baking are good ways of cooking vegetables and proteins. Microwaving vegetables is good too. You don't need to use a lot of water as you do with boiling, and so you don't lose nutrients in the water you drain off. Frying not only adds fat and causes weight gain, but there is some evidence that the process of frying increases exposure to heterocyclic amines that can cause cancer. You have to be careful with grilling or broiling meat too, as the crispy, burned bits at the edges are also thought to cause cancer. Some processed meats (hot dogs, bacon, cold cuts) contain high levels of nitrates. It is suggested that you avoid these in large quantities.

Frozen fruits and vegetables are nutritious too. They are picked at the peak of ripeness and may be a better value nutritionally than fresh produce that is trucked for days or weeks to the final destination. They are often cheaper and easier to find, especially if you live far from a large supermarket. Canned foods can be high in sugar (fruit in syrup, for example), and canned vegetables often have high levels of salt. Occasional use of these products is not harmful. If they help you get your daily quota of fruits and vegetables, they can really be useful because they don't need to be refrigerated.

Food safety is also important. Everything that we eat is potentially the home of many micro-organisms that can and do make people sick. If your immune system is suppressed, you have to be extra careful. Here are some rules to follow.

- Always wash your hands before eating (sing the alphabet song to make sure you're washing long enough and remember to get between your fingers—most people miss that part).
- Wash fruits and vegetables before preparing them to eat.
- Be really careful when handling raw meat, fish, and eggs. Wash your hands before and after handling raw proteins.
- Keep raw meat separate in the fridge and make sure it is wrapped tightly.

- Thoroughly clean all surfaces (cutting boards, countertops) that come into contact with raw meat before and after handling.
- Cook foods to the correct temperature (see www.foodsafety .gov/keep/charts/mintemp.html).
- Keep hot foods hot and cold foods cold.
- Be very careful about eating at buffets. If you are immune compromised, you should avoid these completely.
- Don't eat or drink unpasteurized foods or liquids (e.g., honey, cheese, milk).
- If you live in the country and use well water, you may want to get the water checked by local authorities to make sure it is safe to drink.

Being *overweight* has been linked to cancer recurrence. Most of the studies about this have been done in older men and women, so we're not sure if they apply to young adults. Strict dieting is usually not recommended for cancer survivors because of the risk of loss of muscle mass that often occurs with very restrictive diets. Following the guidelines for a healthy diet will often cause gradual and safe weight loss for those whose eating patterns are less than perfect. A diet focused on fruits and vegetables, whole grains in moderation, small amounts of proteins, and even less fat will cause a healthy weight loss for most people. Following the U.S. Department of Agriculture and Health Canada's Food Guide is healthy and balanced. If you do want to lose weight, talk to your healthcare team and a nutritionist or dietitian for advice and support.

I had a healthy lifestyle before, and the doctors said that one of the better things to do for everyone is to stay healthy. So when things happen like this, your body can recuperate. My doctors have also said that I've been able to recuperate faster than those that I started

with because of the healthy lifestyle I had before. I re-
ally do appreciate the fact that my mother taught me
how to cook. And that I taught myself how to cook. So
I source all the food that I eat. I eat only what I can.
I'm living in a diabetic family as well. I've learned
how to drink coffee black and not have lots of sugars.
                        —Jomar, acute lymphoblastic leukemia

Do you need to take supplements? If you watch TV or read magazines, it would seem that the answer is "yes!" Up to one-third of newly diagnosed people start taking supplements. But research suggests otherwise. There is NO evidence that taking supplements is helpful for cancer survivors. It does not prevent recurrence or improve survival. There is evidence that for some kinds of cancer, taking vitamin E supplements actually increased mortality. Those who smoke or drink alcohol are at increased risk for negative outcomes if they take beta-carotene supplements (Rock et al., 2012). If your diet is balanced, you do not need to take extra vitamins or minerals.

Many people are interested in taking *antioxidants* because of the publicity about oxidative stress in tissues as a result of cancer and as a side effect of treatment. Fruits and vegetables are a great source of naturally occurring antioxidants including vitamin C, vitamin E, and carotenoids. Many supplements contain higher than the recommended daily doses of these antioxidants, and if you take them while on treatment, they may interfere with the effectiveness of the treatment. There is still much to be learned about this topic. Until there is good evidence to support guidelines, it is suggested that cancer survivors avoid dietary supplements that contain more than 100% of the daily recommended dose unless your oncologist specifically prescribes otherwise.

Can you drink alcohol? It all depends on the kind of cancer you have, whether you are a man or woman, and if you are in active treatment or recovery/remission. Cancers of the head and neck are associated with the use of alcohol, and continuing to drink may increase your risk of recurrence or of a second cancer. Alcohol is processed through the liver and can cause inflammation of that organ, so drinking during treatment can interfere with the metabolism of chemotherapy agents. And, in turn, chemotherapy and radiation therapy cause inflammation of the liver, so drinking alcohol may cause additional symptoms. Alcohol can also irritate the lining of the mouth and throat, so if you have stomatitis or dry mouth, you may want to avoid it. People who've had head and neck cancer are at a fourfold risk of developing a second cancer if they drink as little as two drinks a day. Very little research has been done on alcohol use and cancer survivors, especially young adults.

How much water should you drink? Your total fluid intake every day should be about

- 15 cups (3.75 quarts or 3.5 L) for men
- 11 cups (2.75 quarts or 2.7 L) for women.

Depending on what you eat, about 80% of your water intake comes from foods. If you drink 8–10 glasses of fluids every day, you should have no problem meeting your body's needs. If you have diarrhea or vomiting, you have to be vigilant in replacing lost fluid. Many symptoms that people with cancer experience, such as dry mouth, bad breath, fatigue, nausea, and light-headedness, may be a sign of dehydration.

What's the take-home on diet and nutrition?

- There's no magic diet that can cure cancer or prevent recurrence.
- A balanced diet with high-quality nutrients can help you heal from treatment, avoid obesity, and fight off infection.
- Keeping well hydrated can improve your daily quality of life.

Exercise

I've tried to take an active role in finding ways to make my life a little easier, a little bit healthier. I definitely follow all of the advice of my doctors. I'm not trying any alternative medicine, not any vitamins or any supplements or stuff like that, but I keep as active as I can. I walk a lot and I've done a little Pilates. I've started going back to the gym moderately, just using my cardio machines, mostly stretching, but not a lot of weights because of where my pain is.

—Naomi, Hodgkin lymphoma

It is widely accepted that physical exercise plays an important role in recovery from cancer treatment. Moderate exercise can improve fatigue (even if that sounds contradictory), reduce depression, increase self-esteem, and boost endurance and muscle strength. It almost sounds too good to be true, but it really is! Studies have also shown that for certain kinds of cancer (breast, colorectal, ovarian, and prostate cancer) and usually in older adults, regular exercise reduces the risk of recurrence and improves survival. Regular exercise reduces the risk of getting cardiovascular disease, diabetes, and osteoporosis in the general (non-cancer) population and is thought to do the same for cancer survivors. This is important, as some of the long-term effects of cancer treatment cause these conditions.

In an overview of 56 trials with 4,826 participants, moderate to vigorous exercise was found to improve health-related quality of life and reduce anxiety, fatigue, and sleep disturbances in all cancer survivors other than women with breast cancer. Improvements were seen in role functioning, emotional well-being, and physical functioning (Mishra, Scherer, Snyder, et al., 2012). In another review of 40 studies of exercise including a total of 3,694 participants, various kinds of exercise (strength and resistance training, walking, cycling, yoga, Qigong, and tai chi) showed improvements across a wide range of outcomes including body image, sexuality, sleep disturbances, fatigue, emotional well-being, pain, anxiety, and social functioning (Mishra, Scherer, Geigle, et al., 2012). This is powerful evidence, and based on many studies, there has been widespread acceptance of the role of exercise in improving outcomes for cancer survivors.

According to the American Cancer Society, the American College of Sports Medicine, and the Centers for Disease Control and Prevention, the following are recommended for all cancer survivors.

- Some form of exercise five times a week
- Warming up for 5–10 minutes before walking, swimming, or cycling
- Maintaining moderate intensity for 30–45 minutes per session
- Cooling down for 5–10 minutes after exercising

> *I do have a fairly physical job. And when the weather allows me, I will be first guy out on the front street with my kids and a football. That's about as far as I go with that. And I take them to the park as much as I can. But I'm not the guy in the gym. I just don't have time. I don't have enough minutes in the day as is.*
> —*Brian, leukemia*

To do any kind of exercise, you need to find something you actually enjoy. It can be really helpful to find someone to exercise with because it is easier to say no to yourself than to your exercise partner. Be realistic about what you can or should be doing. Your capacity may have been significantly affected by your treatment, and you don't want to hurt yourself or become frustrated; that will just lead to avoidance in the future. If you have never exercised, start slow and gradually increase intensity and frequency.

> *I'm fortunate enough to live in an apartment where we have a small gym. And even if it's the slowest kind of walking that I can do on our machines, I do that. We have an elliptical. I purchased, I don't want to call them grandma weights, but the very lightweight bracelets that you buy at the store and unfortunately that's all I could lift, but every little thing counts. And it's just continually telling yourself that your health is dependent on you. If you do nothing, you get nothing. If you do just a little bit and you stack them all up, then you'll get something.*
> *—Jomar, acute lymphoblastic leukemia*

What kind of exercise you can do depends partly on what treatment you had, your health, and the presence of side effects. For example, if you're having radiation, you should not swim in chlorinated pools because this can irritate your skin. If you are anemic, you should delay exercise until that is corrected and your energy levels are better. If you are immune compromised, you should avoid team sports and gyms to reduce your exposure to germs and viruses. If you usually exercise, you may want to cut down on your intensity while on treatment. There's no reason why light exercise cannot be done while undergoing chemotherapy or radiation (surgery may require a break for four to six weeks). Talk to your oncology team about what you can and cannot do.

It's a good idea to consult with a knowledgeable sports therapist or trainer before you get back to exercise if you stopped or if you've never exercised. They need to have an understanding of the effects of cancer and its treatment and how this may influence what you can and cannot do. Although pushing yourself to work hard while exercising can be good, you also don't need to injure yourself. An informed trainer can help you get maximum benefit while reducing risk. Some cancer centers have rehabilitation programs that include a physical exercise component. This is great because you don't have to explain your cancer; they will know what you need and will help you set safe goals for yourself. Check out your local YMCA; they may have special programs for cancer survivors. It can sometimes be a challenge to find a program that is not mostly old(er) people. The fact is that older people make up most of the survivorship population, so you may be the only young(er) person in the class or the gym. Research suggests that exercising as part of a group rather than alone is more likely to be successful. The group may hold you accountable to be there for your regular sessions, and if you miss, someone may call you to see where you are and how you're doing. And you are more likely to be competitive in a group than on your own.

Not everyone loves to exercise or enjoys physical exertion (or sweating!). Many forms of exercise are gentle on the body and are a great place to start if you are a beginner. Yoga has been studied in breast cancer survivors and has been shown to decrease stress, anxiety, and depression. Resistance training such as lifting weights or using resistance bands has also been shown to have positive effects on muscle strength and stamina. A combination of aerobic activity, resistance exercise, and yoga may be the perfect recipe for regaining health and wellness after cancer.

Everything kind of hit from the surgery and the stress,
to the fact that I went from living life at like 120 km

an hour to being completely off work. I'm a girl who runs marathons. I go to the gym four or five times a week and am super active, and I could barely walk around the block when I got home. I wasn't allowed to run. I wasn't allowed to exercise. I could walk for, at first, five to ten minutes a day. I'd get up and eat breakfast and shower, and I'd have to go lie down. This was so unbelievably different from what I was used to. All I wanted to do was work out and go to work. And I couldn't do those things.

—Alison D., kidney cancer

The 411 on Exercise

- Do something, anything, physical for just 10 minutes. You'll be surprised at how easy it is to keep going.
- Use music to inspire and challenge you as you exercise. Upbeat music can really get you going (or try something quieter for yoga or stretching).
- Start small with something you know you can do, and progress slowly but surely.
- Take friends or family members with you for company and for their health.
- Get a dog—they have to get out a couple of times a day.
- Remember that exercise counteracts fatigue. So, being tired is not an excuse.

Complementary Therapies

Complementary and alternative medicine (CAM) therapies refer to services, products, and practices that are not considered part of conventional medicine, according to the National Center for Complementary and Alternative Medicine (http://nccam

.nih.gov/health/whatiscam). This organization describes five kinds of complementary therapies:

1. Mind-body therapies, such as music therapy and guided visualization
2. Biologically based therapies, such as supplements
3. Manipulative and body-based therapies, such as yoga
4. Energy therapies, such as therapeutic touch and Reiki
5. Alternative medical systems, such as acupuncture or homeopathy.

Many cancer survivors use these kinds of therapies over the course of their cancer journey. In one study, almost 57% of women with early-stage breast cancer used at least one kind of CAM, most often supplements (Wyatt, Sikorskii, Wills, & Su, 2010). Most people regard the use of vitamins and other supplements as pretty mainstream and not all that alternative, so for the purposes of the following section, we will focus on the other four types of CAM. People use CAM to enhance physical and emotional well-being, to improve their health, to take back control of their health after treatment, and to prevent recurrence (Habermann et al., 2009), but we really don't know if any of these therapies actually work. The research in this area is still in its infancy, and studies are not common in all areas.

Mind-body therapies such as guided visualization and music therapy have been used for a long time as a way of decreasing distress and anxiety in people with cancer. In one study on guided visualization and acupuncture, participants experienced improved quality of life compared to a control group. They also reported less fatigue and less loss of appetite, as well as increased emotional health and decreased anxiety (Sawada et al., 2010). Participants were encouraged to visualize their bodies as healthy, strong, and free from whatever symptom was bothersome to them at the time. Guided imagery may be particularly useful for those who experience anxiety and nausea related to chemotherapy because they can practice it during treatments.

Music therapy has also been shown to help patients relax. One study of younger adults suggested that two hours of music therapy (listening to music, singing, and playing an instrument) can increase relaxation and decrease heart rate (Chuang, Han, Li, & Young, 2010). Another study of patients with breast cancer found similar results (Chuang, Han, Li, Song, & Young, 2011). However, it was not clear from either study how frequently music therapy needs to be done or for how long. For younger people (ages 15–25), listening to music may be particularly helpful. It is well known that for people in this age group, listening to music is an important part of life in general. When people with cancer in this age group were asked about the role that music plays in their lives after diagnosis, they described it as providing supportive messages and allowed them to find meaning in the cancer experience. Music allowed them to visualize positive emotional and physical scenarios that were of benefit when they were going through stressful treatments. It also enabled them to connect to others in a supportive way (O'Callaghan, Barry, & Thompson, 2012).

Manipulative and body-based therapies such as yoga may be helpful, particularly for women with breast cancer. In a study of women with breast cancer undergoing radiation therapy, positive results were experienced, including less sleep disturbance, less fatigue, and better social and physical functioning (Cohen, 2005). A review of 13 studies of the impact of yoga, mostly involving patients with breast cancer, showed large reductions in depression, anxiety, and distress, moderate reductions in fatigue, moderate increases in general social and emotional health, and increases in overall quality of life (Buffart et al., 2012).

Yoga is often done together with meditation and relaxation. Therefore, research showing the benefits of yoga may be confounded by the influence of meditation. In a review of 10 studies of yoga with a total of 762 participants, yoga was shown to improve aspects of psychological health including anxiety, depression, distress, and stress (Lin, Hu, Chang, Lin, & Tsauo, 2011).

Based on the evidence from these reviews, yoga may be of benefit to cancer survivors of all kinds. It is important to start this practice with appropriate supervision. Like any kind of exercise, your instructor should be well trained and knowledgeable, not just about yoga but also about the effects of cancer and cancer treatment on the body and mind. Yoga by definition is not a competitive sport, and although initially you may not be able to do any or all of the poses well, or even at all, persistence will pay off. After time you will notice the benefits in improved emotional well-being, physical flexibility, and strength. But it's not a race. Take it slow and easy,

Energy therapies such as therapeutic touch and Reiki have also been used for a long time in patients with cancer. Therapeutic touch involves the provider consciously directing energy exchange by placing his or her hands over the survivor's body (not actually touching the body) for 10–20 minutes. The theory behind this is that our energy extends a few inches beyond the physical body, and when we are ill or stressed, the free flow of energy over the body is interrupted. Therapeutic touch is thought to increase the flow of energy and restore it to its normal state. This CAM therapy has been studied in people with cancer and has been shown to reduce pain and anxiety and help with relaxation (Coakley & Barron, 2012). Reiki (the practice of a special kind of touch) has existed for thousands of years. There is limited evidence to support its use, but it is widely practiced and recommended despite this. Research into its effectiveness in patients with cancer is very limited. Despite only a small number of studies into these kinds of therapies, people with cancer are often very interested in trying them (Hart, Freel, Haylock, & Lutgendorf, 2011). They are seen as noninvasive, nonthreatening, and relaxing.

Alternative medical systems such as acupuncture or homeopathy are popular among cancer survivors. Acupuncture uses the insertion of fine needles in specific places on the body to correct an imbalance in the body's energy. The traditional form of acupuncture, called Traditional Chinese Acupuncture (or TCA), is based on a diagnosis of "imbalance." Western Medical Acupuncture (or WMA), however, uses acupuncture techniques to treat medically diagnosed conditions (Choi, Lee, Kim, Zaslawski, & Ernst, 2012). This may appear to be a subtle difference, but it is a difference. Reviews of published studies on the use of acupuncture in patients with cancer suggest that although there is some evidence to support its use for treating chemotherapy-induced nausea and vomiting, further research is needed to assess its use in treating other symptoms (Garcia et al., 2013). However, another review suggests that acupuncture can safely be used to treat a number of treatment-related symptoms including pain, dry mouth, fatigue, insomnia, hot flashes, anxiety, and depression (O'Regan & Filshie, 2010).

Homeopathy involves ingesting highly dilute solutions of various remedies. It is based on the principle of "like cures like": highly dilute formulations of substances that cause symptoms of disease in healthy people are thought to cure people who are ill. This CAM therapy has traditionally been used by people with cancer to increase their ability to fight off infection, to improve physical and emotional well-being, and to reduce pain (Milazzo, Russell, & Ernst, 2006). It is controversial, and many people scoff at it as being implausible and not based on sound scientific principles. But in some studies, participants with cancer have noted improvements in fatigue and quality of life (Rostock et al., 2011). Critics suggest that this is purely a placebo response because it is impossible for such dilute quantities of anything to make a difference. Still others suggest that it is safe and may be effective and that further research is needed (Frenkel, 2010). Proponents suggest that homeopathic remedies trigger the body's defense system, but they cannot explain how they do this, and so their effectiveness is questioned. As with all treatments, if it sounds too good to be true, then it probably is, and caution should be used.

If you do choose to see a complementary or alternative therapist, you should ask some questions first.

- What credentials do you have, and where are they from?
- How many people with my kind of cancer have you seen?
- How long have you been in practice?
- How will you decide if your treatment is helping me or not?
- How long will your recommended treatment take?
- What will this cost, and is it covered by insurance?
- Do you earn money for any supplements or products you suggest?
- What studies have been done on the treatments you are recommending for me?
  - Were they approved by an ethics review board, and have they been published?
  - Will you provide me with these published results? If not, why not?

Websites About Complementary and Alternative Medicine

- **National Center for Complementary and Alternative Medicine:** http://nccam.nih.gov

- **National Cancer Institute:** www.cancer.gov/cancertopics/cam
- **Memorial Sloan-Kettering Cancer Center:** www.mskcc.org/cancer-care/integrative-medicine/about-herbs-botanicals-other-products

What Comes Next?

This chapter has discussed the benefits and risks of various strategies to help maximize health both during and after treatment. While some interventions (healthy diet and exercise) are safe and effective, others may be questionable or not based on scientific evidence. The attitude of survivors is often that if something may be able to help, even without supporting evidence from research, why not try it? Most of these interventions are not covered by health insurance, so the biggest impact may be on your bank balance. But if you are interested, ask your friends and family members and even your healthcare team for personal recommendations.

Whatever you try, it is really important to tell your healthcare team what you are doing or taking in the form of supplements or homeopathic remedies. Even something that is "natural" may interact negatively with traditional medication or treatment, and your healthcare team needs to know about it. This is not a Big Brother thing but is important for your safety and also is an opportunity to educate and inform practitioners who may not know about alternative or complementary forms of treatment.

References

Buffart, L.M., van Uffelen., J.G.Z., Riphagen, I.I., Brug, J., van Mechelen, W., Brown, W.J., & Chinapaw, M.J.M. (2012). Physical and psychosocial benefits of yoga in cancer patients and survivors, a systematic review and meta-analysis of randomized controlled trials. *BMC Cancer, 12,* 559. doi:10.1186/1471-2407-12-559

Choi, T.-Y., Lee, M.S., Kim, T.-H., Zaslawski, C., & Ernst, E. (2012). Acupuncture for the treatment of cancer pain: A systematic review of randomised clinical trials. *Supportive Care in Cancer, 20,* 1147–1158. doi:10.1007/s00520 -012-1432-9

Chuang, C.-Y., Han, W.-R., Li, P.-C., Song, M.-Y., & Young, S.-T. (2011). Effect of long-term music therapy intervention on autonomic function in anthracycline-treated breast cancer patients. *Integrative Cancer Therapies, 10,* 312–316. doi:10.1177/1534735411400311

Chuang, C.-Y., Han, W.-R., Li, P.-C., & Young, S.-T. (2010). Effects of music therapy on subjective sensations and heart rate variability in treated cancer survivors: A pilot study. *Complementary Therapies in Medicine, 18,* 224–226. doi:10.1016/j.ctim.2010.08.003

Coakley, A.B., & Barron, A.-M. (2012). Energy therapies in oncology nursing. *Seminars in Oncology Nursing, 28,* 55–63. doi:10.1016/j.soncn.2011.11.006

Cohen, L.E. (2005). Endocrine late effects of cancer treatments. *Endocrinology and Metabolism Clinics of North America, 34,* 769–789. doi:10.1016/j. ecl.2005.04.008

Frenkel, M. (2010). Homeopathy in cancer care. *Alternative Therapies in Health and Medicine, 16*(3), 12–16.

Garcia, M.K., McQuade, J., Haddad, R., Patel, S., Lee, R., Yang, P., ... Cohen, L. (2013). Systematic review of acupuncture in cancer care: A synthesis of the evidence. *Journal of Clinical Oncology, 31,* 952–960. doi:10.1200/ JCO.2012.43.5818

Hart, L.K., Freel, M.I., Haylock, P.J., & Lutgendorf, S.K. (2011). The use of healing touch in integrative oncology. *Clinical Journal of Oncology Nursing, 15,* 519–525. doi:10.1188/11.CJON.519-525

Lin, K.-Y., Hu, Y.-T., Chang, K.-J., Lin, H.-F., & Tsauo, J.-Y. (2011). Effects of yoga on psychological health, quality of life, and physical health of patients with cancer: A meta-analysis. *Evidence-Based Complementary and Alternative Medicine, 2011,* Article ID 659876. doi:10.1155/2011/659876

Milazzo, S., Russell, N., & Ernst, E. (2006). Efficacy of homeopathic therapy in cancer treatment. *European Journal of Cancer, 42,* 282–289. doi:10.1016/j. ejca.2005.09.025

Mishra, S.I., Scherer, R.W., Geigle, P.M., Berlanstein, D.R., Topaloglu, O., Gotay, C.C., & Snyder, C. (2012). Exercise interventions on health-related quality of life for cancer survivors. *Cochrane Database of Systematic Reviews, 2012*(8). doi:10.1002/14651858.CD007566.pub2

Mishra, S.I., Scherer, R.W., Snyder, C., Geigle, P.M., Berlanstein, D.R., & Topaloglu, O. (2012). Exercise interventions on health-related quality of life for people with cancer during active treatment. *Cochrane Database of Systematic Reviews, 2012*(8). doi:10.1002/14651858.CD008465.pub2

O'Callaghan, C., Barry, P., & Thompson, K. (2012). Music's relevance for adolescents and young adults with cancer: A constructivist research approach. *Supportive Care in Cancer, 20*, 687–697. doi:10.1007/s00520-011 -1104-1

O'Regan, D., & Filshie, J. (2010). Acupuncture and cancer. *Autonomic Neuroscience: Basic and Clinical, 157*, 96–100. doi:10.1016/j.autneu.2010.05.001

Rock, C.L., Doyle, C., Demark-Wahnefried, W., Meyerhardt, J., Courneya, K.S., Schwartz, A.L., ... Gansler, T. (2012). Nutrition and physical activity guidelines for cancer survivors. *CA: A Cancer Journal for Clinicians, 62*, 242–274. doi:10.3322/caac.21142

Rostock, M., Naumann, J., Guethlin, C., Guenther, L., Bartsch, H.H., & Walach, H. (2011). Classical homeopathy in the treatment of cancer patients—A prospective observational study of two independent cohorts. *BMC Cancer, 11*, 19. doi:10.1186/1471-2407-11-19

Sawada, N.O., Zago, M.M., Galvão, C.M., Cardozo, F.M., Zandonai, A.P., Okino, L., & Nicolussi, A.C. (2010). The outcomes of visualization and acupuncture on the quality of life of adult cancer patients receiving chemotherapy. *Cancer Nursing, 33*(5), E21–E28. doi:10.1097/NCC.0b013e3181d86739

Wyatt, G., Sikorskii, A., Wills, C.E., & Su, H.A. (2010). Complementary and alternative medicine use, spending, and quality of life in early stage breast cancer. *Nursing Research, 59*, 58–66. doi:10.1097/NNR.0b013e3181c3bd26

CHAPTER 9

Psychosocial Support

As you have read (and lived), a diagnosis of cancer and the treatment that follows changes life forever. But this does not mean that life after cancer is worse. In fact, it can be better—or at least different in a good way. Cancer certainly changes what is normal, and most of us want our lives to be normal, or whatever "normal" means to us. One aspect of the cancer experience that is very important is support, not only from parents but also from peers, including others with cancer whom you meet along your cancer journey. This chapter will describe what young adults have reported about their needs for social support, where they find or create it, and the importance of peer support.

Coping With Cancer

I was so unhopeful in the very beginning of hearing the talk of the statistics and my situation and how the cancer had developed in me and all that kind of stuff. All those numbers piled on me and I felt useless and that I was never going to make it. And my mom stopped and said, "You know what, the doctors have not told you that you have a date to live to." That, to her, meant that I was going to recover, and there was no doubt in their mind either that I wasn't going to make it. So she was the confidence that I didn't have that I could rely on 24/7.

—Jennifer, acute myeloid leukemia

Any change in one's life requires adaptation or coping. Yes, you can stick your head in the sand and refuse to accept the changes, or you can adapt. In reality, nothing in life is static. We change and adapt on a daily basis. But being forced to accept a new reality and altered health requires effort and mental flexibility. One of the important tasks when faced with illness is coping effectively. How you cope can have far-reaching and very real effects on your emotional health. This in turn can affect your physical health; they're connected.

Although there are many things that you can't do because of cancer, how you choose to respond to the disease is under your control to a certain but very important extent. You cannot change the fact that you have cancer, but you can modify or alter your response to the cancer (the same goes for people who are annoying or hurtful: you can't change them but you can change your response to them!). How you choose to cope with cancer is modifiable. You can choose to cope negatively (not a great idea), or you can choose to cope effectively. The point is to reduce the amount of distress you experience as a result of the disease.

I always poke fun of my cancer. Other people feel awkward when I tell them what's happened to me. But I joke around with them and say, "Hey, I'm the one with it; you don't have to worry about it." To make light of it I guess. Things happen. That's how you do it.

—Jomar, acute lymphoblastic leukemia

He (my now-husband) always made fun of me, not in a bad way, but he always said that he wanted the fun girlfriend because I had a wig and I was one of the people who always wore my wig. I never took the wig off in public. And obviously at home I did. But so I wouldn't kiss him or make out with him with the wig on because it would mess it up. So he said, "I want the fun girlfriend. I want the bald girlfriend because that's when I'm allowed a good deal."

—Melinda, breast cancer

The 411 on Effective Coping

The following coping styles are associated with reducing distress.
- Having an internal (personal) locus of control—believing that you are in control of your life and not blaming others when bad things happen
- Having an optimistic outlook—making the best of situations
- Using a minimizing approach to situations—not blowing things out of proportion
- Having a fighting spirit—meeting challenges head-on
- Being problem-focused—analyzing what is facing you and working on finding a solution
- Seeking social support—reaching out to others

You have to take each day as it comes because every day is different. When you're having a good day, take advantage of it. When you're having a bad day, real-

ize that it's a bad day and let people know so that they can be prepared. But take that day for yourself as well. Taking it as it comes is how I did it. I don't think there was another way that I could have done this. Maybe smiled or laughed more, but I don't think there's anything I could have done differently.

—Jomar, acute lymphoblastic leukemia

The 411 on What NOT to Do

The following coping styles are thought to be destructive and may increase distress.

- Avoidance—the opposite of being problem-focused
- Denial—this may work in the short term but has poor long-term consequences
- Wishful thinking—this is connected to denial and avoidance; not focused on reality
- Being resigned to whatever happens—the opposite of having a fighting spirit
- Blaming yourself—this is not productive, period.

The Positive Impact of Cancer

Cancer can have some benefits. Please don't throw this book out the window after reading that statement. A study of more than 500 adolescents and young adults with cancer reported some interesting findings (Bellizzi et al., 2012). The researchers looked at both positive and negative outcomes of having cancer and divided the people into three groups according to age: 15–20, 21–29, and 30–39. All three groups reported positive changes to relationships with mothers, future plans and goals, and confidence in taking care of one's own health.

Those in the oldest group (30–39) reported a positive effect with their relationship with spouse or partner (70%); this was greater than those in the other two groups (60%). Almost half of all groups reported that they had a more positive attitude toward life goals, and more than 50% of those in the study reported that cancer had a positive effect on their religious or spiritual beliefs.

The Downside

Cancer definitely has a negative impact on various aspects of life. The same study that reported positive effects of cancer also reported a number of negative effects. Around 60% of all three groups said that the cancer caused them to have a poor body image. Almost half of all respondents said that cancer left them feeling out of control with their lives. About a third said there was a negative outcome on their plans for work, and two-thirds also reported a negative impact on their financial situation. While the majority reported a positive outcome on their spousal or partner relationship, 25% of everyone in the study stated that the effect on their partner relationship was negative, and 50% reported a negative effect on their plans to have children. Those aged 20–29 and 30–39 also reported a greater negative effect on sexual functioning than participants in the 15–20 age group (58% vs. 40%).

So what does this study tell us? In a nutshell, there are good and bad sides to cancer, as there are to most things in life. You can weigh them against each other, and everyone will come up with a different take-home message. How you respond to the good and the bad is dependent on many factors, including previous experience dealing with adversity, your general outlook on life (optimist vs. pessimist), and how you deal with challenges. What this study tells healthcare providers is that cancer has a global and far-reaching effect on young adults and that they have many and varied needs for support.

Location, Location, Location: Treatment Setting and Getting Your Needs Met

Depending on where you receive care, your support needs may be met or may go unmet. Reading about this may be frustrating because often you don't know what you're missing or what services you could have accessed if only you knew where to find them or were even offered them. Cancer care can be provided in large multidisciplinary cancer centers with special departments that offer psychosocial care, rehabilitation, support groups, patient education libraries, Internet access, and other services and amenities. They will often have age- and tumor site–specific clinics. These types of treatment centers usually are located in large cities and often have a high profile and good reputation. If you live close to one of these and are referred there, you are likely to get cutting-edge treatment with lots of support. If you live in a rural or remote area, your care may take place in a private oncologist's office or a small hospital with limited support services. This restricts your access to on-site supportive care and may mean that unless you go searching for information and support, you might not hear about what is available to you.

> *A lot of people are shy, and when you have an illness, you feel very isolated from everybody else. But when you get up on that ward, you talk to people you never thought you would talk to. And you talk to them like they're your own family. You become your own fami-*

ly up on that ward. And you give each other sugges-
tions. Throughout the day you talk about how your
night went, what happens, this and that, and how
you dealt with it.

—*Brian, leukemia*

Some young adults are treated in pediatric clinics rather than adult settings, or follow-up care may take place in pediatric clinics because that is where it started years ago and your doctors want to continue seeing you (they love seeing their successes!). This can feel really weird, and not just because of the child-friendly wallpaper and art on the walls. However, one study found that young adults treated in pediatric settings were more likely to have their needs for mental health services met and also to receive information about fertility (Zebrack et al., 2013). This study also found that young adults had unmet needs for information about diet and exercise. Surprisingly, the participants in this study did not use the Internet for information gathering or support (see more about this later in the chapter).

Other studies suggest that support needs are high for young adults, particularly for support from others who are going through cancer. Those who have "been there and done that" appear to be more useful than friends who do not have cancer (Zebrack, Ganz, Bernaards, Petersen, & Abraham, 2006). This may be due partly to the gap between someone who is dealing with the physical and emotional challenges of cancer and those without the disease, but it also may be because their usual developmental tasks have been halted. Many young adults are dependent on their parents because of their cancer and are not doing the same things as their healthy peers, such as attending college, working, and so on. People who have been through similar experiences are able to empathize with you in a real way, while your friends without cancer may remind you constantly of how your life has changed, which may bring you down (Goodall, King, Ewing, Smith, & Kenny, 2012).

> *I had a lot of support from people that had gone through this before me. A guy had gone through it and it really helped to see somebody standing in front of you that had just gone through it and they're looking OK. That was huge. That was a big mind settler for me.*
>
> —*Brian, leukemia*

Young adult cancer survivors are known to experience greater distress than older adults. So, if you are seen in a treatment center where there are mostly older adults, your needs for support by healthcare providers may not be met. Young adults report that they need help understanding and figuring out the best way to manage issues related to insurance; this kind of help may not be offered if the rest of the patients are older and do not have the same need (Zebrack & Butler, 2012). In addition, young adults with cancer have said that they need help talking to their children about the cancer, and support for this may not be provided in an older adult care setting.

> *I waited a longer period of time before I reached out for additional help. And after going through it, I was quite surprised on how supportive and helpful it was for me. I don't think I would have done it earlier, but you have to go at your own pace. The only other thing I can think of to tell someone else going through this is to really dig deep into your soul, because you're probably stronger than you think you are.*
>
> —*Jennifer, acute myeloid leukemia*

If you've had a delay in diagnosis after being told over and over by healthcare providers that you are too young to have cancer and are eventually diagnosed later, and possibly with more advanced cancer, you are likely to not trust the healthcare system. This can affect information seeking because once trust is broken, it can be really hard to believe what you are told after that. Healthcare providers who are patronizing or critical about the young adult's choices (for example, missing an appointment to go to a social event) are also not trusted (D'Agostino, Penney, & Zebrack, 2011).

It's About Me: Self-Efficacy

It's OK to cry. It's OK to be mad. But you still have to get up every day. And you still have to take care of your kids. And still you have to take care of yourself. You have to take care of yourself before you can take care of anyone else.

—Robyn, breast cancer

Believing in your ability to manage your cancer is known as *self-efficacy*. As you've grown older and matured, you have probably experienced this in other aspects of your life. Having self-efficacy in the context of cancer has been shown to improve quality of life (Zebrack, 2009). Interventions to increase self-efficacy include support groups and educational programs. Seven factors are thought to constitute self-efficacy in cancer (Merluzzi, Nairn, Hegde, Sanchez, & Dunn, 2001, as cited in Zebrack, Hamilton, & Smith, 2009). How many do you have?
1. Maintaining activity and independence
2. Seeking and understanding medical information
3. Practicing stress management

4. Coping with side effects from treatment
5. Maintaining a positive attitude and accepting the cancer
6. Regulating emotions
7. Seeking support

Many of these factors are benefits of joining and attending support groups, in person or online. So, let's talk about support groups.

All in the Pool, Together: Support Groups

It is generally accepted that support groups are good for you. Some healthcare providers can be quite insistent that you go to a support group and keep going, for your own good. Some people really like them and get a lot of benefit from them. Others don't like them at all and would rather walk on hot coals than go once, and certainly not a second time. It all depends.

I joined the Younger Women's Peer Support Group. Amazing. They're all in current treatment. So I met with women who were a little bit behind me. I met women who were a little bit ahead of me. I met women that were right where I was. And it was those women that I bonded and connected with and was really able to get answers and feel as though I could spill my guts to. Sure, I had friends. I had family. But unfortunately, they just have no clue. It was that group of women that I found the connection to get through where I was at that point.

—Aimee, breast cancer

Different kinds of support groups exist, and one or more may be suitable for you at different points along the way.

Cancer type specific: This kind of support group is intended to bring together people with the same kind of cancer of different ages and stages. For example, a breast cancer support group would include women of different ages who have had cancer diagnosed at different stages and have had different kinds of treatments, but they all have been diagnosed with the same kind of cancer.

Age specific: A support group for young adults is age-specific. The support group may be exclusive to those between the ages of 20 and 30, for example. Group members will have different kinds of cancer but all will be of a similar age and will presumably have similar challenges and concerns based on their stage of life.

Educational in focus: These support groups are intended to provide participants with information about a specific topic such as coping with a cancer diagnosis or preparing for chemotherapy. They usually have a formal agenda and include information sharing rather than mutual support.

Affectively oriented: These groups focus on helping participants cope with distressing feelings or losses. The intent is to help those attending deal with their emotions and learn from and support each other through difficult times.

Is This the Right Group for Me?

I connected with Young Adult Cancer Canada and went to my first retreats and met other people. It was just this huge, life-changing experience. I've been able to meet some really wonderful people and have some really amazing, amazing experiences because of that. Through that whole process, it was just telling your story over and over again. But then also realizing that a lot of the things that you're feeling or experiencing or concerned about, you share with other people

*your age, which is really hard. Because I lost a lot of
friends because of my cancer experience . . . that isolation that you get from feeling disconnected from everybody else. That your experience in life is so completely
different. So I think that was always there on an un-
spoken level.*

—*Cheryl, cervical cancer*

Some people are joiners; they like to be part of a group and
will "jump into the pool" feet first. Others are more careful and
want to know more about the group, what is expected of participants, and what will happen at meetings. It is helpful to ask
the following questions before going to a meeting.

- Who runs the group? Is it peer led (someone with cancer or
  their spouse/partner), or does a professional (for example,
  a social worker or nurse) lead the group?
- What is the focus of the group—support, education, or emo-
  tion/coping?
- Who is the facilitator? Is it a professional, or do group members take turns to lead the group?
- What is the makeup of the group? Are partners and family
  members welcome?
- What is the format of the meeting?
- Do I have to pay to attend?

There are no right or wrong answer to these questions, but
this information can prepare you for what happens, or you may
want to look for another group if you don't like what you hear.

The Good Things About Support Groups

Attending a support group is a good thing for many people,
and perhaps even more so for young adults with cancer who
otherwise will have few peers going through the same or similar experiences.

> *It's nice to sit in a room and know that almost everybody else in that room has an idea of what you're going through. Because I don't ever feel like that, at other times. Even though I haven't fully processed it yet, I don't feel like my friends and my colleagues really understand. It's nice to be around people who can relate to having had cancer at any age, but they (a young adult group) can worry about being single and about dating, or having children or the possibility of having children, or jobs, because we're not at an age where we can take early retirement or where there's all sorts of sick time or other stuff built up.*
>
> —*Alison D., kidney cancer*

Young adults with cancer have reported the following benefits from participating in support groups.

Meeting peer survivors: This is very important, as forming friendships is a key task of young adulthood and your "healthy" friends will have little or no experience of cancer at this age.

Being able to talk about your cancer experience: Cancer should not happen to young people. Your friends may not know what to say to you, and you may be censoring what you tell them. Being with others in similar circumstances allows you to talk freely, ask questions, and learn from others about how they cope with cancer.

Letting it all hang out: Participating in a group with your peers allows you to express yourself freely, without the fear of upsetting your partner, parent, sibling, or friend. Young adults who go to support groups say it is the only place where they can say exactly how they feel without the need to censor themselves to protect the feelings of loved ones.

Feeling "normal": Having cancer can be an isolating experience, but being with others in a similar place in their lives can help you to feel like you are normal within the group, rather than being different from everyone else who doesn't have cancer.

Learning about new or alternative treatments: Even though other people's treatment regimens may be quite different from yours, you may hear about other medications that are being used and how others cope with common side effects. You can use this knowledge to start a conversation with your healthcare team about whether any different or newer treatments are available that could help you.

Helping others: Being part of a support group can give you the opportunity to assist your peers, especially once you have gained confidence in your own coping skills. This can feel really good; helping others (altruism) makes us feel worthy, and we can all use some of that!

> *It was really good to connect with other young adult cancer survivors who understood. And even that for me was a bit stressful, going to my first retreat. Because I thought, "I'm going to go and these are all going to be people who've been really sick and they've had to go through chemo and radiation and they could potentially die." And I went, and I didn't feel that at all, which was so good. And I think I realized that everybody has different experiences. But in terms of the overriding themes, the feelings, the things that happen, there's just more similarities than there are differences. And it was just so nice to connect with people. And to realize that you're not completely crazy.*
>
> *—Cheryl, cervical cancer*

The Other Side of the Coin: Some Cautions About Support Groups

Not everyone loves public forms of support. Support groups may not meet your needs or may make you feel uncomfortable. Before you decide that *all* support groups are not for you, think about what it is that you don't like about the thought of a support group. Attending a support group can have some downsides.

- Seeing others who are sicker than you or have a recurrence can be scary and depressing.
- Hearing negative experiences can increase your anxiety.
- If you feel pressured to share your feelings and are not ready to do that, it can feel intimidating.

But many studies report that overall, the advantages of being part of a support group outweigh the disadvantages, and a skilled facilitator can help members to cope with all of the above negative feelings.

Hooray for the Internet!

There has been huge growth in the availability of online support groups in recent years. This has been very important for a number of reasons.

- It provides options for those who live far from major centers and have fewer opportunities for face-to-face support groups.
- They also help those who have limited transportation or who are not feeling well enough to go out.
- They usually don't limit the number of people who can participate. With larger numbers of people participating, you are more likely to find someone with the same cancer as you who is of a similar age.
- Online support groups also feel safer for some people; you can lurk and learn without feeling pressured to speak out.

- You can also take your time in thinking about what other people have posted and provide a thoughtful response instead of just blurting out what's in your head.
- Some support groups use Skype™ or programs that allow participants to see each other during online chats.

> *My online support group . . . I didn't find it until after cancer. I wasn't very active online during cancer because you do research and pretty much everything you find tells you you're going to die. So I look at things now and I'm so glad I didn't look at that when I was going through treatments. But I found my support group afterwards and it was pretty amazing. It's a young survivors' support group for women. The age range is 20 to 50 basically. And they're just amazing women. I'm about 5½ years out from cancer now, and my three best friends that I see regularly are from there now. The online support group is still a lifeline that I have. And I like to give back, and I think that it's pretty amazing to have that support group because they understand me more than anyone else in my life can because they've been there and done it.*
>
> *—Melinda, breast cancer*

What's Out There?

A large number of support groups are available that are specifically for young adults or adolescents. Some are U.S.-based; others are from Canada or other countries. Take your pick—go to the websites and learn what is available and how you can benefit from one, some, or many!

- **Camp Mak-A-Dream** (for young adults and teens): www .campdream.org
- **First Descents** (ages 18–39): www.firstdescents.org
- **Living Beyond Breast Cancer** (has a conference, C4YW, for young women with breast cancer): www.lbbc.org
- **Next Step** (for those up to 40 years of age with various life-threatening illnesses): www.nextstepnet.org
- **Prepare to Live** (ages 18–40): www.preparetolive.org
- **Stupid Cancer** (ages 15–40): www.stupidcancer.org
- **Teen Impact** (ages 13–30+): www.teenimpactprogram.com
- **Teens Living With Cancer** (ages 13–22): www.teenslivingwith cancer.org
- **Ulman Cancer Fund for Young Adults** (ages 15–35): www .ulmanfund.org
- **Vital Options International** (ages 18–40): www.vitaloptions.org
- **Young Adult Cancer Canada** (ages 15–39): www.youngadult cancer.ca
- **Young Survival Coalition** (ages 15–40 with breast cancer): www.youngsurvival.org

> *I will say those two experiences (cancer conferences) have helped me heal a lot because you get to talk to people that are your same age and going through the same issues. You get to cry with and complain to them. And you can kind of let your guard down. You don't have to be strong for them because they're going through the same thing.*
> —*Robyn, breast cancer*

What Comes Next?

There are many ways to find support, and to support others in return. This feels good and can help you learn how to cope based on how others who have "been there, done that" have managed. Remember that you don't have to commit to anything forever. Dip your toes in the support pool and see if the water feels good. The next chapter will talk about dealing with family and friends, a sensitive topic for many.

References

Bellizzi, K.M., Smith, A., Schmidt, S., Keegan, T.H.M., Zebrack, B., Lynch, C.F., ... Simon, M. (2012). Positive and negative psychosocial impact of being diagnosed with cancer as an adolescent or young adult. *Cancer, 118,* 5155–5162. doi:10.1002/cncr.27512

D'Agostino, N.M., Penney, A., & Zebrack, B. (2011). Providing developmentally appropriate psychosocial care to adolescent and young adult cancer survivors. *Cancer, 117*(Suppl. 10), 2329–2334. doi:10.1002/cncr.26043

Goodall, S., King, M., Ewing, J., Smith, N., & Kenny, P. (2012). Preferences for support services among adolescents and young adults with cancer or a blood disorder: A discrete choice experiment. *Health Policy, 107,* 304–311. doi:10.1016/j.healthpol.2012.07.004

Zebrack, B. (2009). Information and service needs for young adult cancer survivors. *Supportive Care in Cancer, 17,* 349–357. doi:10.1007/s00520-008-0469-2

Zebrack, B.J., Block, R., Hayes-Lattin, B., Embry, L., Aguilar, C., Meeske, K.A., ... Cole, S. (2013). Psychosocial service use and unmet need among recently diagnosed adolescent and young adult cancer patients. *Cancer, 119,* 201–214. doi:10.1002/cncr.27713

Zebrack, B., & Butler, M. (2012). Context for understanding psychosocial outcomes and behavior among adolescents and young adults with cancer. *Journal of the National Comprehensive Cancer Network, 10,* 1151–1156. Retrieved from http://www.jnccn.org/content/10/9/1151.long

Zebrack, B.J., Ganz, P.A., Bernaards, C.A., Petersen, L., & Abraham, L. (2006). Assessing the impact of cancer: Development of a new instrument for long-term survivors. *Psycho-Oncology, 15,* 407–421. doi:10.1002/pon.963

Zebrack, B., Hamilton, R., & Smith, A.W. (2009). Psychosocial outcomes and service use among young adults with cancer. *Seminars in Oncology, 36,* 468–477. doi:10.1053/j.seminoncol.2009.07.003

CHAPTER 10

Family and Friends

Any parent will tell you that the worst thing that can happen in their lives is for one of their children, no matter how old, to get sick. It doesn't matter if they are all grown up with children of their own; for a parent, that is the very worst. So when a child is diagnosed with cancer, it's as if the bottom of their world has just dropped out and nothing will ever be the same again. For siblings, life changes too, no matter how old they are and how the relationship was before. Your friends will also be affected by your diagnosis. Cancer changes everything for them, too—what was once certain is no longer certain, and often people just don't know what to do.

> *Most dads don't really cry a whole lot. My dad is no exception. This made him cry. To see me in the hospital those first couple of days . . . I can see a lot of anguish. When I went to my chemo treatments, they would always send someone with me and, again, making sure that I wasn't going through this alone because it can be very isolating and a lonely experience. They've been huge. Like letting me live in their house for six weeks when I got out of the hospital. They cooked and cleaned for me. All I had to do was*

165

just make sure I got out of bed every morning and took my medication, and they would help take care of the rest. Because they didn't want to leave me because they saw how strong and how independent I was in the years leading up to it and suddenly there I am in the hospital bed, on the verge of death.

—Serena, non-Hodgkin lymphoma

In children, illness occurs in the context of the developmental milestones that they have achieved. When teenagers get sick, their parents are still the legal guardians. In all likelihood, they are still living in the same home as their parents, and the parents have financial and functional responsibilities for them. Young adults are supposed to move out and begin lives of their own, independent of their parents. For young adults who have a partner or spouse, their emotional attachments to their parents are altered and their primary emotional focus shifts to the partner relationship. This is how it should be. It's not that young adult children no longer love their parents; it's just that the love changes with time and maturity. Some parents and their young adult children describe their relationship as a friendship with less emphasis on emotional and functional support and greater equality.

I have a good relationship with my mom, and it's still really stressful. I've lived on my own for about six or seven years now, so moving back, it's like, you've changed and you've had a lot of experience in your life since leaving home, but my mom still kind of treats me like I'm a child and doesn't quite get that I've been taking care of myself for a long time and that I can. She still thinks that I need a lot of taking care of.

—Naomi, Hodgkin lymphoma

With age, sibling relationships also change. However, one's place in the chronologic order of the family does not change. Older siblings are often seen as the caretakers of younger brothers and sisters; younger siblings often retain their "baby of the family" status long after they have grown up. And middle children, no matter how old they are, often feel like they have to fight for attention from their parents. Serious illness in any sibling threatens the natural order of these relationships and puts their traditional roles in jeopardy.

Serious illness also shakes the foundations of your friendships outside your family. Most young adults live under the canopy of the three I's: invulnerability, immortality, and invincibility. Life-threatening illnesses happen to older people, not to their friends and peers. Cancer surprises us all and calls into question just how invulnerable, immortal, and invincible we really are. Many young adults have never experienced death or even serious illness in anyone close to them. When this happens to someone close to them in age or relationship it can be shocking. This shock may translate into their response to your diagnosis.

This chapter will highlight the effects of your diagnosis and treatment journey on your family and friends. It also will provide guidance on how best to give and receive support and how to maintain or create appropriate boundaries. You may want to suggest to those close to you that they read this chapter even if they don't want to read the rest of the book.

"Mom, Dad, I Have Cancer": Disclosing Your Diagnosis

The love that parents have for their children is, in most cases, unconditional and the kind of love that would cause them to jump in front of a runaway train if you were in its path. To hear that you have cancer is a life-changing moment for them. Their immediate response is likely to be disbelief followed by deep sorrow and shock. Just as your life will never be the same, neither will theirs. Parents often say that they would rather have cancer than see their child of any age go through this experience. Their first instinct may be to protect you and to take over, just as they would have done when you were much younger. You may not mind this; it can be comforting to have someone else make decisions for you when you are feeling overwhelmed and stressed. On the other hand, this can make you feel like a small child and may make you angry or pull away from them.

> *I no longer feel like they'll not care if I'm not around. So I'm not just fighting for myself now; I'm also fighting for them. And I will not quit with that on, with that help, with that support.*
>
> —Daylan, B-cell leukemia

There is a natural tension or balance in the relationship between young adults and their parents related to dependence and independence. As you get older, your reliance on them lessens and you are much more independent, even if you live at home or rely on them for financial support. Being sick changes that balance; you may be dependent on them for some things but still want to make decisions about your health and treatment. They may not see it that way. Every cell in their body wants to protect you, and they may try to make you more dependent (or less independent) without realizing what they are doing. To maintain a healthy relationship with them, you have to work this out before sparks fly and angry words are said. They are just reverting to an earlier way of parenting—and you may be surprised to find that you like being taken care of—but you need to set limits of what they can say and do as it relates to your care and decision making.

> *My mom was with me every single day, two to three times a day. So knowing that she would be there the next morning or the next lunchtime was what made me feel happy to wake up and have a plan and be excited to see her. And she was pretty hard on me. So if I didn't want to do my daily jobs, which were necessary to make me stronger throughout the whole hospital stay, she made me do them. And she was never negative and never worried for me. She was the positive light in everything. And it was that tiny hopeful voice in the back of my head at the same time. When I told her I was diagnosed with AML on the phone, she immediately said, 'You'll get through this.' She didn't have one ounce of doubt.*
>
> —*Jennifer, acute myeloid leukemia*

Parental Responses 101: The Three H's

Helpless: Some parents are so shocked that they have no idea how to help you or themselves. They may even seek support from you instead of the other way around.

Hovering: Some parents go into protective overdrive. They become hypervigilant and treat you like you are three years old and incapable of independent thought or action.

Helpful: Some parents become superstars of support and are there for you in the best ways possible.

You will have to deal with whatever their response is, but you can also choose to not respond. There will be times and situations where your best response to them is to create some distance so that you can do what you need to do without the pressure and stress of worrying about them or keeping their anxiety under control. Here are some potential responses to the three H's.

Helpless: I need you to support me (and my partner) right now. If you cannot do that, I will have to find that support elsewhere, and that may make you feel bad. This is happening to me/us and I/we don't have the energy to support you.

Hovering: I know you mean well, and probably can't help it, but I am an adult, and this is happening to me. Your response is overwhelming me right now. I know you want to protect me, but I am actually feeling stressed and pressured by your attention. Please give me some space to process what is happening.

Helpful: Thank you.

> *My mom is a fixer. She just tries to go on and on and distract you from your problems and say, "This works for me, so obviously it's going to work for you," and "This is what you should do." I told her last week, "Mom, I know you mean well and I know you're trying, but just say 'this sucks,' just agree that this really sucks and say 'I'm sorry.'" She's trying, she's really trying, and I'm trying to talk to my brother more, and at some point I'm probably going to have a sit-down conversation with my dad.*
>
> *—Alison D., kidney cancer*

For some parents, and also other family members, your diagnosis is so terrifying that they become avoidant or prefer to live in denial. This can feel invalidating and frustrating, but we all have different ways of coping. If your family is not providing you with the kind of support you need, ask for it. If they can't support you after that, you may have to find support somewhere else. Or they may just need time to figure out what to do and how to be there for you. Cancer can and often does bring families closer—but not always.

> *I used to have a closer relationship with my father than I did with my mother. And once all this cancer stuff happened, it switched gears and I started talking to my mother more than my father. I think the fact that it has to do with my breasts kind of creeps my dad out a little bit. As soon as he found out, the first thing that he did was hop on the Internet and start researching everything there was about breast cancer, because that's something that he felt he could do. If he couldn't be there to talk about the girlie parts, he could be there to talk about the science and make sure that I'm getting the best treatment possible. So that was cool.*
>
> —*Sarah, metastatic breast cancer*

Your family and friends may think that if they provide you with information, such as from magazines, television, the Internet, friends, and acquaintances, you will be grateful and will act on that information. This may be anything but helpful. The information may not pertain to your kind of cancer and may be useless at best and harmful at worst. The best way to deal with this is to thank them and tell them that your healthcare providers are doing their best to treat you the most effective way they can.

Family Radio: What Not to Tell and What to Tell

You need to discuss with your parents what they can share about your illness with others in their social group or with extended family members. In some ways, having a young adult child who is ill feels like having a small child who is ill, and back then they could share stories about your fever or chicken pox far and wide. But this is *your* cancer, and you have control over what they tell and to whom. You need to make this clear at the outset. They should ask permission to share any information about you to anyone, including your siblings. If they aren't the kind of people who would ask permission, you should tell them up front what they can say and what they cannot share *before* they break your confidence or confidentiality.

In the same vein, they may assume that your healthcare team will share information about your diagnosis or treatment plan with them, and they may be hurt or angry to discover that by law this information cannot be shared with them without your permission. The following U.S. laws and documents are there to protect your privacy. (Canada has similar laws, but they may be different depending on the province that you live in.)

- The Health Insurance Portability and Accountability Act (HIPAA) of 1996 protects the sharing of your health information with anyone.
- A Health Care Power of Attorney is a document that allows you to specify someone else to make healthcare decisions on your behalf if you cannot speak for yourself.
- An authorization to release personal information is a document that allows your healthcare team to release information to someone who you want to know about your health and treatment plan.

It is strongly advised that you have a conversation with the person or people you choose for these functions. You may think that your family knows what you would want to happen if you cannot speak for yourself, but they may not. This can cause them a great deal of stress as they try to figure out what you would want. The most helpful instructions you can give them are detailed and clear. The following are some questions (among many others) that you may want to consider.

- Do you want to be placed on a ventilator if you cannot breathe on your own? For how long?
- Do you want to be fed by tube or IV if you cannot eat or drink?
- If you are in a coma and you get an infection, do you want to be treated with antibiotics?

This is difficult stuff to think about and plan for. Hopefully no one will have to make these kinds of decisions—not you, not your loved ones, not ever. But you do need to be prepared, as these are impossible topics to address when you and they don't know your wishes.

> *I don't know if it was like fight-or-flight for me. It probably was, because I thought, "You know what, I'm not letting you give up." And her feet were so burnt and so puffy that I made her get up. I made her go for a walk. I didn't realize how uncomfortable it was for her. I just thought that if you sit in this bed and you lie in this bed and you don't do anything, you will die. You will die. You will just say, "I'm done. I'm leaving." And I couldn't have that.*
>
> —Gayle, mother of young adult with
> acute myeloid leukemia

Siblings Are Special

> *[My other children], they've got their own families. They weren't as good as I would have liked them, but that's me; I'm very family orientated and they're maybe not. So, when she got really sick, I would phone them and say, "You know what, you need to come now*

because J's really sick. She's really sick and you need to
come and see her now because I don't know that she's
going to make it." So they were really good and came.
But, like I said, they have their own families. And I
don't think they really got it. I don't think they really
got the fact that she might die.

—*Gayle, mother of young adult with*
acute myeloid leukemia

No matter what kind of relationship you have with your siblings—good, bad, or indifferent—there is a special bond between you. Your cancer will turn their world upside down, and
it is often difficult for them to find support for themselves. Your
parents are focused on you and themselves as they try to figure
out how to cope with your cancer. Your siblings may get lost in
the chaos. It is not unusual to see siblings revert to a previous
way of functioning (or not functioning) at times of family stress
such as this. Long-forgotten grievances and attitudes may rear
up, and old jealousies (for parental attention, as an example)
may appear again. While it is your cancer and you are the one
going through tests and treatments and eventually learning to
live a new normal kind of life, your siblings may act as if you
are doing this deliberately to cause them pain. This may not
make sense in the moment, and it is not a rational and mature
response but is suggestive of their panic and confusion. On the
other hand, your siblings may respond in the most helpful and
supportive ways, perhaps surprisingly.

Your siblings know your parents as well as you do and can act
as a buffer if they are hovering or helpless. They can support
your parents as they support you. They can be there for your
partner or spouse and can be just what your own children need
most when they could use some support. But if you have a con-
flicted or difficult relationship with your siblings, it may be bet-

ter to have very little expectation that they will step up and be helpful or supportive to you. Not all families grow closer in the face of serious illness; some just become more fractured and have more stress and tension. Your siblings may not be able to express their feelings and instead appear to withdraw from you. There is virtually no formal support for siblings, especially if they are young adults like you. In many ways, they are the forgotten ones in your cancer journey.

> *And we (my husband and I) both looked at each other and said, "We're not going to be mad at each other. We know we're going to be under a lot of stress. We know things aren't going to go the way we want, but we're not going to take it out on each other." We actually verbalized that to each other. And we both said that to each other out loud and we made an agreement that, no matter what happens, we will not take it out on each other because, you know, you always want to blame somebody when there's stress involved. So we knew from the past stressful issues that we had to do that. And that was the best thing we ever did because maybe in the last three years, maybe once or twice we, you know, yelled at each other over silly things. But we both made that promise to each other we wouldn't allow it to affect us as a couple.*
>
> —*Susan, mother of young adult with*
> *metastatic breast cancer*

Friends Indeed

I just thought, these are not people that I can connect with anymore, that I have anything in common with. We see the world so completely differently that . . . in a big way I envy them. I think it's great if you can sit there with your happy little subconscious denial of death. Great. But I just don't belong to that club anymore. It's hard enough dealing with everything else and then to have to try and explain myself to people who I didn't feel were making an effort to understand. So it was really good to connect with other young adult cancer survivors who understood.

—*Cheryl, cervical cancer*

As difficult as it is for your family to see you ill, it is also difficult for your friends to see you confronted by cancer. Like you before cancer, they think that they are invulnerable, invincible, and immortal. Many adolescents and young adults take risks—this is a normal part of growing up. And most of you have managed to escape untouched by those risks. This fuels the belief that you are invulnerable and invincible. Young people generally have little fear of death because that is something that usually doesn't touch you at your age. Those of you who have experienced the death of a friend from an accident or suicide know the shock and disruption that such a loss causes. Hearing that a peer has a serious illness often has the same effect.

Considering how young we are, and how little experience we have knowing someone with cancer—they've been pretty awesome. They try and include me. There's always a little tinge of a bit of disappointment when I see pictures or something on Facebook of an event that happened with a bunch of my friends and I know I haven't been invited because I

have cancer, and they probably were like, "Oh, Nao-
mi probably can't come to this or wouldn't want to
do this" because it involved something that they as-
sumed does not coincide with cancer, like staying
out late or sleeping out or something like that. But
they're probably right; I probably wouldn't feel that
comfortable doing those things anyway, but it's nice
to be asked. But I still see them a lot, and they invite
me—a lot of them live in the city and they do come
up to the suburbs to see me once in a while. And peo-
ple call to check in and leave me messages.

—Naomi, Hodgkin lymphoma

Some of your friends will meet the challenge alongside you. They will offer to drive you to appointments or run errands for you. They will try to drag you out to the bar or a movie thinking that some distraction will help you to escape reality for a while. They will feed and walk your dog and offer to play endless video games with you. These kinds of friends are worth their weight in gold. But others may disappoint you; they will run away as soon as the going gets rough. Decline an invitation to a ballgame with them, and they interpret it as a rebuff and will not ask again. Much like potential dates, do you want to spend time with someone who can't accept that, right now, a movie or drink is the last thing you want? This can be painful for you, especially if you supported them through a hard time of their own. Often the more vulnerable that people feel, the more likely it is that they will distance themselves or even flee from contact with you. If friends have never faced adversity personally, they may not know how to act, and you may not feel like teaching them this lesson. Letting a mutual friend know that you are hurt or disappointed in their behavior may help, as the message can be passed along.

Some of my friends that I hadn't seen for a long time came out of the woodwork and really were supportive. And some of them didn't want to talk about it. I don't know if they were scared . . . . And some of the people around me I notice even now, they're jealous of the attention I got from it, but it's not attention I sought or wanted at all. I think everyone has their own ways to deal with it. Everyone has their own ways to deal with grief and death and dying. But then you have to let them deal with it how they need to deal with it.

—Robyn, breast cancer

The one thing that I do notice, though, not just with my friends, but everybody, is that nobody can understand. They think, "Oh, you had cancer, but you didn't die and now you're back at work, so you're OK." But they don't understand the daily struggle that I used to wake up to in the morning and how the GVHD [graft-versus-host disease] affects me.

—Graham, leukemia

If There's Anything I Can Do . . .

Some of my friends that I would talk to, they didn't want to hear me be sad; they didn't want to hear me express what I was scared of. I remember we were all at a pub, we were just talking, and one friend being absolutely appalled that another one of my friends and I were having a conversation about the fact that I could die. And later on, the friend who was very appalled by it was like, "I can't believe that you're talking about that, why are you putting that out there that that could happen?" Some people [would say], "You have to think only positive things. I'm not going to talk to you unless it's positive." A couple of friends were a little bit more receptive if I was up to talking that day, just listening and not really saying anything.

—Alison D., kidney cancer

Friends and family members often say, "Is there anything I can do to help?" and that's where the conversation ends. You feel overwhelmed with what you have to do, should do, or can do, and you just shrug. You may also want to do more than you are able to and therefore don't ask them to do anything. They may be cautious about overstepping the boundaries that you have created for yourself and don't know what they can or should do. You may have to be proactive in letting them know what you need and want them to do. Some suggestions:

- Practical things around your home such as laundry, cleaning, watering houseplants, walking the dog, cleaning out the cat litter, shopping, paying bills, emptying the garbage, or sorting the recycling
- Helping you organize drivers to get you to and from medical appointments
- Informing friends and family members about your progress (clear instructions about what can be shared and what should be private are vital here)
- Getting you books from the library and taking them back by their due date
- Downloading movies and music for your music player or tablet

- Helping your parents with household chores so that they can spend quality time with you

What Comes Next?

Your family and friends can be a great support system for you through your cancer journey. They know you best and care about you. But they can also interfere and be a source of stress for you when you least need it. Some people say that when faced with cancer, we become more of who we really are, deep down inside. The same could be said for your family and friends—the good ones will get better, and the bad ones may be best left by the wayside. Bottom line: there are no rule books for this for anyone. Most people act instinctively at first and then, with time, in a more measured and thoughtful way. The next chapter deals with going back to work or college, essential steps in the cancer survivorship journey.

SECTION III. Being an Adult

CHAPTER 11

Return to Work and School

W ork is a reality of adult life. Love it or hate it, at some point most or all of us have to get a job and go there on a regular basis. Work is one of the hallmarks of being an adult. For many, preparation for work involves going to school (such as a college or university) for some length of time. Work/education is important and fulfills many social and financial needs. It is also important as a marker of normalcy during and after a cancer diagnosis. In this chapter, you will read about the function of work or school in daily life and the challenges that cancer presents to young adults. You will also learn some strategies to help you in returning after taking time off for treatment.

> *Some days I have really good days, and some days it's just tough to get through the day because my energy goes up and down. And to balance work with all the hospital appointments and stuff, it's tough. People ask me, "How are you doing? What are you up to?" And I say, "Well, you know, I'm a full-time employee and a part-time patient."*
>
> *—Graham, leukemia*

Why Is Work or Studying Important?

Despite sometimes being a drag, work or studying has important benefits in our daily life.

1. It provides us with a sense of self-identity.
2. It's a sign that life is normal again (or close to normal).
3. It provides meaning and significance to life.
4. It provides financial rewards.
5. It provides a role in family life and structure.
6. It provides us with social interaction.
7. Doing well at work or school has benefits to self-confidence and self-image.

> *I feel guilty not working. I feel like [my husband] is making the money and paying the bills, and I'm not contributing to that aspect. I want to work but I don't know what I want to do. But then, at the same time, I'm trying to just balance that. So to return to work even just part time is not even something tangible right now in my life. I can't even think about getting up to go to work for a whole entire day and then come home and make supper and do all the things that are your normal life. It wouldn't fit in right now with me, as much as I want it to happen. I have to just take one thing at a time, and eventually I'll get there.*
>
> *—Jennifer, acute myeloid leukemia*

If you're lucky, you have a job or field of study that engages you. What does this *engagement* mean? Work engagement is defined as the positive experiences at work that are fulfilling and lead to vigor (high levels of energy and the willingness to invest in work activities), dedication (sense of inspiration and pride in what you are doing), and absorption (being happy at work and involved in what you are doing so that time goes by quickly) (Schaufeli, Salanova, González-romá, & Bakker, 2002). If you are engaged in your work or studies, you are less likely to quit and are more likely to strive to do better. If going to work or school has all of these benefits, it is not hard to see how going back to work or school after cancer has meaning beyond getting a regular paycheck or getting credits toward a degree or diploma. For many, work also provides health insurance, and this is very important when dealing with cancer. Young adulthood is a time when education and the work you do have a large influence on future earnings and work potential. Cancer causes an interruption in these plans, and many are highly motivated to get back to work or their studies. Unfortunately, not all work or studying is engaging. If you feel bored with or disconnected from what you do, it may be tempting to give up or not go back. But let's start with the positive. What helps cancer survivors in returning to work or school?

You *Can* Go Back

Most young adults with cancer do go back to work or school. In one study, 72% went back within 15–35 months (Parsons et al., 2012). But going back may require some accommodations on the part of your employer and school, and you have a part to play in that, too.

The 411 on Going Back to Work or School

- The less intense the treatment you had, the more likely you are to be able to return to work or studying.
- It is important to be realistic about the requirements (such as workload and duties and course load) and your abilities.

- An occupational health expert can provide guidance on accommodation in the workplace and what you can do to work smarter (not harder).
- Your work supervisor or school counselor/adviser can be an important ally in helping you deal with colleagues as you transition back to work or school.

I think health also has to deal with mental health, and I was getting very sad with staying home and not being around people. With higher precautions needed at work, I've moved my cubicle farther away from people. I'm still around them but farther away. And I'm taking part-time work right now. Having an employer that really cares about your well-being is important. Not only do I have good benefits, but it comes hand in hand with the person and the company that's employed you and the ability for them to accommodate and understand.

—*Jomar, leukemia*

Accommodations to the workplace may include flexible work hours, being able to rest when you need to, having a place to rest that is quiet and comfortable, changes to your duties or responsibilities, or changes to the physical workspace to enable you to do your work. Accommodations for college may include reducing your course load, seeking assistance from disability services to arrange for longer time to write exams or do laboratory work, getting help with reading and with writing papers, using voice-activated dictation software for writing papers, or recording lectures instead of taking notes. But what if you can't go back to work because you have lingering side effects of treatment that affect your ability to go back to your previous work or to find a new job?

Why Do Cancer Survivors Not Return to Work/Studies?

Cancer survivors are 1.5 times more likely than healthy adults to be unemployed (de Boer, Taskila, Ojajärvi, van Dijk, & Verbeek, 2009), and 50% report some problems in the workplace (Parsons et al., 2012). There are many reasons why going back to work or school may be problematic. Some are related to the cancer and its effects, whereas others have to do with the workplace and the specifics of the work itself. Some are modifiable and some not.

> *I had savings before, so I was in pretty good shape. I had to apply for a stop in my [student loan] payments, so they've given me six months, and I'm sure I could reapply for that if I need to. I'm trying to just create a little nest egg so that when I do have to go back to work and I have to move back, I'm not scrambling to pull the money together. And hopefully I have a job waiting for me when I get back. That's the plan; I think that's what we're all saying.*
>
> —Naomi, Hodgkin lymphoma

- Cancer factors
  - Age at diagnosis: The older you are, the less likely you are to return to work (this obviously relates to older adults more than young adults).
  - Stage of disease: People with more advanced disease are less likely to return to work or school.
  - Complex and multimodality treatments: More complex treatments make return to work or school less likely.
  - Need for hormone manipulation: Breast cancer survivors on estrogen-modulating drugs are less likely to return to work or school.

- Health status
  - Cognitive impairment (memory and concentration issues)
  - Physical limitations (pain, fatigue, disfigurement)
  - Psychosocial changes (depression, anxiety)
  - Lack of social support
- Work/school factors
  - Type of work (manual labor vs. sedentary)
  - Supportive vs. unsupportive environment
  - Employer's or school's willingness and ability to make accommodations
  - Relationships with peers, coworkers, managers, and supervisors

How you feel about yourself may influence your ability to go back to work or school and to stay there. Feeling negative about your situation and being unable to see a time when things will improve affects your plans for your career (Stern et al., 2010). This is about being a pessimist rather than an optimist. While this is partly a personality trait, you can learn to think in a more positive way about yourself and your situation.

Many cancer survivors require some accommodation in the workplace or at school, and others' responses can have a significant impact on this. If you feel different because you've lost weight or your hair hasn't grown back yet and your colleagues comment on this and treat you differently, you may feel out of place or even stigmatized. You are not likely to stay at work if you feel this way. Much depends on what, if anything, your coworkers were told about your cancer and any absences from work you had to take. If they have been given your responsibilities without an adequate explanation, they may feel overburdened. If you then return and are given special treatment without any explanation, they are likely to feel upset and may take it out on you. It is important that they are given a reason for your absence and return with any accommodations, but how much they are told is up to you and the manager or supervisor who is responsible for assigning tasks.

Protection Under the Law

Laws are in place that protect you once you go back to work. The Americans With Disabilities Act protects workers in workplaces with more than 15 employees, and cancer is regarded as a disease that impairs ability to work. Under the terms of this act, reasonable accommodation must be made for eligible workers as long as this does not pose an undue hardship on the workplace. The employer does not have to provide you with aids to help you do your job better and is not expected to make allowances for lower output. But, you cannot be fired or denied benefits because you have cancer, and the employer must make reasonable accommodations in terms of work hours and allowing you time off for medical appointments. There is a claims process, and cases are decided on an individual basis. People with cancer submit more claims for job loss, unequal treatment, and interpersonal problems than people with non–cancer-related impairments (Feuerstein, Luff, Harrington, & Olsen, 2007), and cancer survivors have been successful in winning their claims. Cancer survivors may feel discriminated against. This discrimination may be hidden (covert) or out in the open (overt). *Covert* discrimination happens when someone is passed over for promotion or denied benefits. It is usually subtle, and your employer may claim that it has nothing to do with your abilities or disabilities. *Overt* discrimination is much easier to recognize. The workplace itself may be hostile, and coworkers or supervisors may make negative comments about you or make threatening actions toward you. The environment may be hostile if reasonable accommodations are not made to help you do your job. For example, if you have to stand at a cash register and the employer will not allow you to sit or will not provide you with a chair, this is overt discrimination and is against the law.

Being able to attend medical appointments is another challenge for those returning to work after cancer treatment. The Family and Medical Leave Act (FMLA) applies to workplaces with more than 50 employees. Under this act, you are allowed to take up to 12 weeks of unpaid leave in a 12-month period to deal with medical issues. You are also allowed to reduce your work hours, and when you do return to work, you must be placed in an equivalent position to the one you left. The employer must also continue to provide health insurance and other benefits while you are away. This act may apply to your partner or parents and enable them to take time off to help you.

Canadians (other than Quebec residents) are covered under Employment Insurance sickness benefits as long as you meet certain criteria. Details are available online at www.servicecanada .gc.ca/eng/ei/types/sickness.shtml#what.

Doing It Right: Going Back to Work

If you ask your oncology care provider when you can go back to work, the most common answer is "When you're ready." But what does that mean? There are many reasons to feel ready— like when your bank balance is nonexistent—but this does not mean that you are physically or mentally ready. You may be mentally ready after months of daytime TV, but you may not be physically ready to do a job that requires stamina and strength. Or, you may be physically ready to go back to school, but you may have problems concentrating in class and studying for exams. Many cancer survivors participate in cancer rehabilitation programs at their cancer center or are referred to one of these programs. They are useful to help prepare you for your return to work or school and focus not just on the physical aspects of rehabilitation but also on emotional and vocational aspects as well.

Occupational health experts are people who specialize in issues with returning to work or school. They can be very helpful in assessing your readiness to return and in identifying what, if any, accommodations need to be made. Back-to-work/school plans should be made *before* you plan to go back. The occupational health expert will assess your abilities as well as the requirements of your workplace and will make recommendations to maximize your potential for success successful. One of the most helpful aspects of working with an occupational health expert is the creation of a plan for your return to work that you can share with your employer.

A return-to-work plan should include
• The type of work you can do
• How many hours you can work at the beginning
• How those hours will increase over time
• What, if any, accommodations need to be made
• How long the accommodations should be in place (or if they are permanent)
• The date that the plan should be reevaluated
• What information can be shared with coworkers.

What Comes Next?

Going back to work or school is an important marker of your progress from treatment to long-term survivorship. For many, it is the one thing that says "I am myself" and represents normalcy. Hopefully this is a milestone that you have achieved or will negotiate successfully, and being back at work or school will soon feel as though you had never been away. The final chapter in this book deals with participating in research, something that many people with cancer are eager to do or may have questions about.

References

de Boer, A.G.E.M., Taskila, T., Ojajärvi, A., van Dijk, F.J.H., & Verbeek, J.H.A.M. (2009). Cancer survivors and unemployment: A meta-analysis and meta-regression. *JAMA, 301,* 753–762. doi:10.1001/jama.2009.187

Feuerstein, M., Luff, G.M., Harrrington, C.B., & Olsen, C.H. (2007). Pattern of workplace disputes in cancer survivors: A population study of ADA claims. *Journal of Cancer Survivorship, 1,* 185–192. doi:10.1007/s11764-007-0027-9

Parsons, H.M., Harlan, L.C., Lynch, C.F., Hamilton, A.S., Wu, X.-C., Kato, I., ... Keegan, T.H.M. (2012). Impact of cancer on work and education among adolescent and young adult cancer survivors. *Journal of Clinical Oncology, 30,* 2393–2400. doi:10.1200/JCO.2011.39.6333

Schaufeli, W.B., Salanova, M., González-romá, V., & Bakker, A.B. (2002). The measurement of engagement and burnout: A two sample confirmatory factor analytic approach. *Journal of Happiness Studies, 3,* 71–92. doi:10.1023/A:1015630930326

Stern, M., Krivoy, E., Foster, R.H., Bitsko, M., Toren, A., & Ben-Arush, M. (2010). Psychosocial functioning and career decision-making in Israeli adolescent and young adult cancer survivors. *Pediatric Blood and Cancer, 55,* 708–713. doi:10.1002/pbc.22642

CHAPTER 12

Research and Clinical Trials

R esearch is a very important aspect of cancer care. All of the drugs and most nonpharmaceutical treatments exist because of research. Being a participant in a research study is an important way of getting access (without cost) to medications that have not yet been approved, and for some, it is a way of getting really good care at a special treatment center. But research is mostly about doing good for others. Let's start with the different kinds of research that you may be asked to participate in.

What Kinds of Trials or Studies Are There?

Clinical trials involve testing drugs or new ways of giving other kinds of treatment. Survey studies involve people being asked to complete questionnaires to describe their experiences. Some studies involve in-depth interviews in which the researcher asks the participant about what it is like to live with cancer, or to be a parent of a child with cancer, and so on. There are also focus group studies where people with cancer are interviewed as a group and asked specific questions. The reason for these studies is to learn more about the patient or family experience so that healthcare providers can do things better for others in similar situations. Some researchers ask you to fill out questionnaires about your quality of life or level of depression or anxiety before and after some kind of intervention (for example, art therapy, to see if doing art therapy makes a difference for people of a certain age with a certain kind of cancer). These are called *intervention studies*. There are also patient satisfaction surveys in which you may be asked about your experience in the hospital or clinic in order to improve services.

All research involves the participants giving consent to take part in the study, and all research must be approved by various committees before participants can be invited and the study can begin. There are certain instances where the participant doesn't physically sign a consent form, but because they complete a survey or answer questions online or by phone, their consent is implied or assumed. Let's start with a discussion about informed consent and the ethics of conducting research.

"I Do": Consent to Take Part in Studies

And she [the doctor] wanted me to try out this clinical trial. So I asked what was different from the clinical trial than from the treatment I'd be getting? They told me the clinical trial would be a bit more aggressive and there would be different chemos. So I'm like, "OK, I'll try this one first." Maybe it can help me and they can figure out if this works better than the other. So in a way I was helping. And I wanted to do it.
—Daylan, B-cell leukemia

Before researchers can begin any kind of study, they have to get permission from an Ethics Review Board. These usually are associated with universities, although some private companies do this, too. The Ethics Review Board checks to see that the proposed research will be done in an ethical way, that there is no coercion, and that participants' rights are protected. There are international laws about ethical research that state what must be done and what cannot be done to research participants, and the Ethics Review Board ensures that these laws are followed. Members usually include physicians, researchers, nurses, and other healthcare providers as well as lawyers and patient advocates. They cannot be involved in the studies seeking approval in any way. The Ethics Review Board may refuse to approve a study if it does not comply with the ethical standards and laws protecting research participants, or it can ask for changes to the study.

One of the most important issues that the review board looks at is the process of informed consent. All individuals who participate in research must receive enough information about the study so that they can decide if they want to take part or not. The information has to be presented in a way that they can understand, and they have to be able to ask questions about the study and have their questions answered in a satisfactory manner. They should understand that they can withdraw at any time and that their care is in no way influenced by whether they take part in the study. Only after this information is provided should the person sign consent to be part of the study.

Giving your consent to be part of a study or trial means reading forms (often long, complicated, and boring) that explain in great detail what the study is about, the process and monitoring, and what side effects may occur. You are expected to read the forms before agreeing to participate and signing the form. This is often done at a time of high anxiety and distress for people soon after diagnosis, and some agree to be part of a study because they are afraid that if they say no, they will not

196 THIS SHOULD NOT BE HAPPENING: YOUNG ADULTS WITH CANCER

get good treatment or any treatment at all. Some people rush into signing the consent form and then find that they don't remember what they were told and are not happy with their decision to participate at some point in the future (Stryker, Wray, Emmmons, Winer, & Demetri, 2006). It really is important to weigh the pros and cons of taking part and to take as much time as you can to do this. Feeling pressured to sign consent usually leads to regret and dissatisfaction.

Some people don't like the idea of being "experimented on" and so do not agree to take part. Others don't like the idea that they may be in the control group (the group that receives the standard treatment) and will not get a new treatment or won't see any benefit. Others opt to not be part of a trial because this is one of the only ways they feel they have any control at that time, or they may feel that it will take up too much of their time that they would rather spend with family and friends (Quinn et al., 2012). On the other hand, being part of a trial also gives hope to many. For some people, if previous treatments have not worked, this is a way of potentially gaining access to a new treatment that may help them.

But do people really read the consent form and understand what they are reading and agreeing to? A study of bone marrow and stem cell transplant recipients (Shannon-Dorcy & Drevdahl, 2011) suggested that not only do some people not even read the consent properly before signing it, but most (72%) sign it and never go back at any time to check what they had consented to. In this study, more than 90% of the participants had decided that they were going to participate in research even before they were told about any studies. This may reflect the seriousness of the cancer and their desire to be treated, even in an experimental study.

Consent can only be given by someone who has reached the age of legal consent (which varies depending on the country).

For those younger than that, consent is provided by the legal guardian (usually a parent), but the young person should give *assent* where they are able.

In the United States, state and local laws determine the legal age of adulthood; who is legally considered a child may vary from state to state. In most states, 18 is the legal age. State law may also specify circumstances where someone younger than the age of adulthood is legally authorized to consent to medical procedures (for example, in obtaining contraceptive services). In some states, minors can complete the emancipation process and gain certain civil rights, which might include the ability to consent to participate in a clinical trial (U.S. Department of Health and Human Services, 2011).

In Canada, three types of consent forms exist: (1) Assent form for children younger than 16 (with the exception of Quebec, which is 18), (2) Parent/Guardian's Consent for the recruitment of children younger than 16 (18 in Quebec), and (3) Consent Form for Adult (older than 16–18 and mature minors) (Health Canada, 2012).

Checks and Balances

Once the study gets started, the Ethics Review Board may monitor the study to check that the researchers are doing what they said they were going to do. They can stop a study at any point if they find that the researchers have changed something in the study (for example, the kinds of cancers they are studying or how they are asking participants to answer questions). In the case of a study involving medications, the company manufacturing the drug will have its own monitors who check, sometimes without warning the researchers about their visit, to ensure that the protocols are being followed and that the documentation is correct, current, and complete. The Ethics Review Board and the drug company's monitoring committee can stop the trial at any time, for example, if participants are having serious side effects or if the test drug is showing such good results that it would be unethical to withhold the treatment from other people. So let's talk about clinical trials.

What Works? The Purpose of Clinical Trials

The term *clinical trial* usually refers to a study where new drugs are tested in humans to see if they are safe and effective. There are four levels, or *phases*, of these kinds of trials. The new drug may be compared to existing drugs, or the trial may involve trying well-known drugs in different combinations. Sometimes a new drug is tested against a placebo (or "sugar pill"), but this rarely happens in cancer trials, as most cancers need to be treated and to deny someone access to treatment (by using the placebo) would be considered unethical.

Phase 1: These usually involve a small number of patients (often healthy individuals) who are given the drug under carefully controlled and monitored situations in a hospital to see if the drug is safe. They may be given different doses of the same drug to see what side effects occur.

Phase 2: If the drug is found to be safe, the second phase sets out to see if it is effective. In phase 2, a limited number of people with advanced cancer are invited to take part in the study. They may or may not benefit from the drug. This phase is only to see if the drug works. The majority of people who take part in phase 2 studies do not see any improvement in their disease and may experience harmful side effects.

Phase 3: This is the kind of study that most people are familiar with. You may have been or are part of one of these studies. In a phase 3 trial, the new drug is tested against an existing drug to see which is most effective and what the side effects are in a larger group of people. A control group is always used as a comparison (these people get the usual treatment). You have no choice in which group you are placed (see the next section on randomization), and you usually do not know what drug you are getting. Phase 3 trials are often the only way for people to get treatment with new drugs. People who are newly diagnosed are often offered participation in phase 3 trials.

Phase 4: These are postmarketing studies that are conducted after a drug has been approved. Manufacturers are interested in learning about side effects that did not appear in earlier testing, and once thousands or hundreds of thousands of people have taken the medication, these rarer side effects are noticed because so many more people are exposed to the drug. There is usually a way for doctors to report these to manufacturers, who have to report them to the approval agency (the Food and Drug Administration in the United States and Health Canada in Canada). If the effects are serious enough, a warning may be issued or the drug may be removed from the market.

> *A clinical trial is a test run. You're one of the couple people who'll be doing it. They take your results and other people's results and decide if this drug should be used or not. You're the prototype people of what's going on. So I decided to do it. I said, "What the heck. I'm already in a bad place; might as well see if I can get better." So I took this road. And it was aggressive.*
> *—Daylan, B-cell leukemia*

Flipping the Coin:
The Randomization Process

The only way to really know if one drug is better than another is to test it against an established treatment (the control group) without any bias on the part of the research participants or their physicians. To prevent bias, both the patient and the physician must be "blinded" as to whether the patient is part of the experimental group or the control group. The decision about which group you are assigned to is done almost like the flip of a coin (but complex computer programs usually make the choice). Both treatments look the same and are given in exactly the same way, and there is nothing about the appearance of the drug that could tell you if it is the new one or the known treatment. All participants get the same monitoring no matter which group they have been assigned to.

The 411 on Asking Questions About Clinical Trials

The following are some questions you might want to ask about taking part in a clinical trial. They should be included in the informed consent form that you sign, but you may want to ask them anyway.
- Who is funding this clinical trial?
- Why do you think this new drug may work?
- What side effects may happen from the treatment?
- What happens to me if the treatment is harmful?
- What other drugs or treatments should I avoid when I am on the clinical trial?
- Will the results of the trial be told to me?
- Can I get the same drug after the clinical trial is over?
- What are the short- and long-term side effects?
- How do the risks and benefits of the drug compare with available treatments?

- Will costs be covered by the clinical trial (for travel or overnight stays)?
- Will I get paid for being in the study?
- Will this affect my insurance or medical coverage?
- Can study visits happen at the same time as my regular clinic visits?

More information about clinical trials can be found on the following websites.
- In the United States: www.clinicaltrials.gov
- In Canada: www.canadiancancertrials.ca

Should I or Shouldn't I? Risks and Benefits

One of the most important things to remember about taking part in research is that you may not benefit directly from the study. There are certain clinical trials where you will have access to new and experimental drugs and you will not have a chance of being randomly assigned to the control group; this will be clearly explained to you verbally and in written form. If you are not sure, ask before you sign anything or start taking medication. It is highly unlikely that if you are in the control group you would not receive active treatment (that is, you receive a placebo or sugar pill). Once again, ask if you are not sure. It can be difficult to understand everything about what you are being told, especially if you are stressed.

It is very important that the researchers running a clinical trial follow up with all the participants. Each trial starts off with the number of people needed to determine if the new drug or combination of drugs is better than the comparison treatment. So they spend a lot of time and energy contacting participants in trials, often to keep in touch and gather information. You should expect the research nurse to become somebody you hear from frequently, although some people complain that they feel "hounded" by the researchers at times.

The main goal of research is to increase our understanding of health and illness, as well as specific conditions and their treatments. So taking part in a trial may not be about you, but instead about creating new knowledge about how humans experience illness or respond to various treatments. The findings of the research often apply to those who come after you and not directly to you. Taking part in research that does not directly benefit you is a form of *altruism*, doing something for the good of others. Doing something for others is a noble action, and in one study, 47% of those who participated in a clinical trial said that this was an important part of their decision to participate in research, but only 1 in 7 of them reported that their primary reason for taking part in a specific trial was this desire to help others (Truong, Weeks, Cook, & Joffe, 2011). So while the idea was a good one, it was really self-interest that played a larger role in their decision.

Some people agree to take part in a clinical trial because they feel pressure from family members and want to be seen as doing "something." This can be a difficult situation to find yourself in. Your family is telling you to do something, but they may not know the details of what will happen or what the side effects are. Perhaps if they knew this, they would back off. But unless you tell them, they may have a hard time understanding why you don't want to try. Sharing your feelings with them is important because their confusion may go away once they understand the whole picture.

Young adults are often hard to recruit into clinical trials for a number of reasons. Many screen their calls to avoid those from unknown numbers such as a researcher, cancer clinic, or doctor's office. They may change their address and contact information, and the place where they received their cancer treatment may not have accurate contact information for them. Some young adults want to forget about the cancer and avoid follow-up with their healthcare providers.

Perhaps I Should Have . . . : Decisional Regret

Whenever you weigh one option against another—taking part in a trial versus not, trying a new treatment or sticking with the one that your doctor knows a lot about—there is room for second thoughts and regret later. This was discussed at length in Chapter 2 of this book. Regret may occur when you realize that an earlier decision was not the right one and you feel responsible for choosing the wrong thing. Or, you can experience regret when you made a decision under a great degree of uncertainty and afterward think that a different choice would have been better. Finally, you may experience regret in the form of self-blame when a decision you made results in negative outcomes or consequences. When you feel that you had no other choice (for example, you had to join a trial to access an investigational drug), decisional regret may be less likely to occur because you had no other option.

What Comes Next?

Research is an integral part of cancer care, both in providing your healthcare team with the means to treat cancer and prevent it from coming back and for potentially improving quality of life for those affected. It takes a lot of planning on the part of the researchers and could not happen without the generosity of those who choose to participate.

This is the last chapter in the book, but in the following pages of the appendix, you can read about the people who agreed to be interviewed for this book. Their stories may be similar or very different from yours, but we hope you will learn from them.

References

Health Canada. (2012, November 13). Requirements for informed consent documents. Retrieved from http://www.hc-sc.gc.ca/sr-sr/advice-avis/reb-cer/consent/index-eng.php

Quinn, G.P., Koskan, A., Wells, K.J., Gonzalez, L.E., Meade, C.D., Pozo, C.L.P., & Jacobsen, P.B. (2012). Cancer patients' fears related to clinical trial participation: A qualitative study. *Journal of Cancer Education, 27,* 257–262. doi:10.1007/s13187-012-0310-y

Shannon-Dorcy, K., & Drevdahl, D.J. (2011). "I had already made up my mind": Patients and caregivers' perspectives on making the decision to participate in research at a US Cancer Referral Center. *Cancer Nursing, 34,* 428–433. doi:10.1097/NCC.0b013e318207cb03

Stryker, J.E., Wray, R.J., Emmons, K.M., Winer, E., & Demetri, G. (2006). Understanding the decisions of cancer clinical trial participants to enter research studies: Factors associated with informed consent, patient satisfaction, and decisional regret. *Patient Education and Counseling, 63,* 104–109. doi:10.1016/j.pec.2005.09.006

Truong, T.H., Weeks, J.C., Cook, E.F., & Joffe, S. (2011). Altruism among participants in cancer clinical trials. *Clinical Trials, 8,* 616–623. doi:10.1177/1740774511414444

U.S. Department of Health and Human Services. (2011, March 24). What are the requirements for assent and parental permission in research with children? Retrieved from http://answers.hhs.gov/ohrp/questions/7267

The Interviewees' Stories

T his appendix contains abbreviated cancer stories from the young adults and two mothers who were interviewed for this book and whose quotes you have read throughout the text. Not all of them were alive at the time this book went to print, and I hope I was able to express my gratitude to them sufficiently at the time of the interview, as they will unfortunately not read these words.

An author's knowledge of a topic is often not experiential; the author is an expert based on professional experience and book learning. It is the people who "walk the walk" who can "talk the talk." For this reason, I put out a call for young adults to talk about their experience—and was overwhelmed with responses. I interviewed people from across North America, on the phone and in my office. Their stories all changed me and how I see the cancer experience. Their words illustrate and highlight their triumphs, disappointments, compromises, questions, and failures of the healthcare system and healthcare providers. But I could only include truncated quotes from their stories in the chapters of this book, and this felt like I was not telling the whole story of who they are, where they have been, and where they are going.

So I asked the talented Alicia Merchant, who wrote the foreword to this book, to condense their stories as told to me in the interviews. This is what you will read in this appendix—brief stories of those whose words add richness and meaning to the text. I am grateful to each and every one of them.

Aimee

Aimee had been married for five years when on March 15, 2001, at just 29 years old, she felt a pain in her chest. Instinctively, she reached up, and that's when she felt the lump. She knew in her gut that something was terribly wrong. Aimee's mother encouraged her to listen to her instincts and go to the doctor, so Aimee made an appointment with her family physician. He wanted to wait two weeks to see if the lump would shrink or go away on its own. When there wasn't any improvement, things kicked into high gear. Aimee was sent for an ultrasound and a surgical consultation.

What the surgeon saw on the ultrasound alarmed him, and he recommended the lump be removed. Aimee opted to have the surgery, and the pathology results came back positive: Aimee had breast cancer. While waiting for the diagnosis to come in, Aimee and her husband discussed what they would do if the lump was cancerous. Aimee decided that a double mastectomy would be her best option, as she wanted to minimize her risk of the cancer returning. So, Aimee had a double mastectomy along with lymph node dissection, followed by four rounds of chemotherapy. Six months later, she began the reconstruction process.

Aimee has run into some problems with the reconstruction process, but she has never regretted her decision to have a mastectomy. Nor does she regret her decision to have chemotherapy. With a four-year-old daughter and a 15-month-old son, Aimee felt her childbearing was complete, and because her cancer was estrogen receptor–positive, she didn't want to risk exposing herself to the additional estrogen that comes with pregnancy.

Aimee went through genetic counseling and testing to see if she was positive for *BRCA1* or *BRCA2*, known mutations that put certain groups, like Ashkenazi Jews, at a higher risk of being diagnosed with breast and/or ovarian cancer. With a breast cancer diagnosis at a young age and an Ashkenazi background, Aimee was a perfect candidate for testing. It was a frustratingly long year before she learned that her cancer was not linked to any known mutation.

Aimee connected with a peer support group that put her in contact with other organizations that helped to support her and her young family as she went through treatment. Twelve years out from her diagnosis, Aimee no longer does formal peer support as she did in the early post-treatment years but makes herself available to friends and the women in their lives who have received a breast cancer diagnosis. She attends the occasional conference for young women with breast cancer and recently attended a Young Adult Cancer Canada conference where she connected with others in various stages of treatment and wellness.

Alison D.

Alison had a really difficult time just being diagnosed with kidney cancer. The doctors knew that she had a large growth in her kidney, but getting a definitive diagnosis of cancer took some time. It was only after she had surgery to remove the tumor that she knew the diagnosis for sure. This whole time was fraught with anxiety and frustration for her. She didn't know whether she had cancer and so was reluctant to share what she was going through because her friends might think she was being melodramatic. Also, if it turned out to not be cancer, she was afraid her friends would think she was attention seeking. She was worried that the things she was concerned about, like losing her hair if she had chemotherapy, would seem vain and silly. One of her friends told her that it was all right to be scared about that and she wasn't being silly; this seemed to help her cope, but she continues to have problems with anxiety.

During the time that she waited to have the surgery, she buried herself in work. She didn't know what else to do, so she just kept on going and, at times, pushed away family and friends because she didn't want to feel pitied. The surgery itself and the stress associated with the whole process hit her hard. Before this she was a very active person who ran marathons and worked out every day. After the surgery, she had to take it easy, and she got depressed because she couldn't do the things she usually did. Her mother moved in with her for a couple of weeks to help take care of her, which further added to her depression and feelings of helplessness. Although she appreciated the help, it was hard for her to have someone hovering over her, and her loss of independence was a real challenge.

Alison joined a support group, which she found helpful. Talking to people who have gone through a similar experience allowed her to start to process what she has been through. She also sees two therapists, although she does not talk about the cancer to either of them, instead focusing on other issues. Her doctor is optimistic about her chances, but she gets very stressed before follow-up appointments. Fear of the cancer coming back is overwhelming at times, and she worries about not having enough time to do the things she wants to do. The cancer seems to have put enormous pressure on her. She feels as though her life was put on hold, and she is struggling to get back on track, like everyone else around her.

Allison

Allison was 26 and single when she was diagnosed with stage IIb estrogen receptor–positive breast cancer in 2005. With no family history of the disease, the diagnosis came as a shock. She began dose-dense chemotherapy almost immediately, only four days after her diagnosis. Instead of receiving chemotherapy every three weeks, she received it every two weeks. After three months of chemotherapy, she had a bilateral mastectomy.

The mastectomy was the hardest part of the ordeal for Allison. Physically, the procedure caused a lot of pain in her shoulders, arms, and neck, which is still a problem eight years after her surgery. Emotionally, the surgery caused a different kind of pain. Allison would have to disclose her cancer diagnosis and breast reconstruction to future potential partners, and the prospect of that was frightening.

Allison decided the best way to deal with the complications of dating as a cancer survivor was to simply be honest and open about her situation from the very beginning. On her first date with the man who would become her husband, Allison laid it all out on the table. She asked if he had any questions and answered what she could, and they moved on to other topics. When it came close to the time when they would become sexual with one another, her now-husband reassured her that he knew she was uncomfortable with her body but reminded her that everyone has insecurities about their bodies and that the breast reconstruction didn't matter to him. This was revelatory to Allison. This thing that loomed large in her mind wasn't an issue for her partner. He was supportive and loved her for who she was and her body for all it had been through.

In February 2012, Allison and her husband had a daughter, a "miracle baby" given Allison's estrogen receptor–positive breast cancer and her five years on tamoxifen. She and her husband had talked about children before they married, and both knew that she might not be able to get pregnant. Happily, that wasn't the case.

With a cancer diagnosis comes the feeling of losing control. Allison combats this feeling by taking control of what she can by choosing to eat healthily and by using nontoxic cleaning products. She is mindful of what she puts into her body. It's been a long road and a lot of trial and error, but she has figured out an eating plan of lean protein, lots of vegetables, and green drinks that make her feel healthy and strong. By eating healthily, reducing stress, and taking time for her emotional well-being, Allison ensures that she is doing everything in her control to keep her immune system strong.

Though her initial surgery is long in the past, Allison remains an open book about her diagnosis and reconstruction and serves as a mentor to other young women diagnosed with breast cancer. She makes herself available to share her story and answer questions. She has even shown her reconstructed breasts to women facing mastectomy. She knows the long road of breast cancer and does what she can to guide others on the journey.

Brian

Brian began having problems in 2003 when he was 27 years old—little things at first, things he could shrug off or find other explanations for, like weight loss, lack of energy, and recurring infections that needed to be treated with antibiotics. Finally, in 2005, his wife insisted he make an appointment with the family doctor. It took almost four months before he got in to see him, but in January 2006, Brian found himself in the exam room. His abdomen was swollen and hard, and his doctor sent him for an x-ray and blood tests. Later that day, while watching television at home with his wife, Brian got a call from his doctor. His blood tests came back showing an abnormally high number of white blood cells. The doctor wanted Brian to go to the hospital immediately to meet with an oncologist. Brian, his wife, and his mother sat together in an exam room as the oncologist told him he had leukemia. Brian went through more blood tests and was sent home while they figured out the next step.

On his way to the hospital the next day for more tests, Brian felt his ear become plugged. He tried to blow gently to unblock it, but nothing worked. He went in for his exam and mentioned his ear, which didn't concern the doctors at first. That night, however, the doctor herself called Brian and told him something wasn't right with his loss of hearing in his left ear and how high his white blood cell count was. Brian went into the hospital that evening and was immediately admitted to begin plasmapheresis to lower his white blood cell count, one of the highest ever recorded at that hospital. Brian spent a week going through spinal taps, bone marrow biopsies, and treatment, and left the hospital on a number of drugs. Another oncologist asked to take his case on, and Brian accepted. He started Gleevec® (imatinib mesylate), a relatively new drug at the time that they hoped would replace the need for a bone marrow transplant.

Gleevec worked well for Brian, but his oncologist felt that, given his young age, Brian stood to benefit from a stem cell or bone marrow transplant. This would mean blasting his body with high doses of chemotherapy to essentially destroy his entire immune system to prepare it to receive the donor cells. Brian's oncologist explained that the treatment was likely to leave him sterile but that they had the option to freeze Brian's semen for future use. This option proved too costly for Brian and his wife, so they decided to try for another child (they had a five-year-old daughter at the time) before Brian went off the Gleevec for the bone marrow transplant. When Brian went in for his transplant in December 2006, his wife was four months pregnant.

Although Brian's mother was a close match and could have donated stem cells or bone marrow to her son, an unrelated donor was an even closer match, and they decided to go with this choice. Brian was adamant that he would be recovered enough from his transplant to be home in time for Christmas. He forced himself to eat and walk the hallways to build up his strength and energy, and he achieved that goal.

Brian returned to work for the first time since his diagnosis in May 2008. He is fully recovered from his treatment and transplant. His eldest daughter is 12, and his youngest daughter, the one he and his wife call their "wonder baby," is five.

Cheryl

Cheryl and her husband didn't know she was expecting until eight weeks before she was due. She hadn't planned the pregnancy, and it was a chaotic time in her life. Her father had passed away of a heart attack just a month before, and here she was suddenly about to become a mother. Little did Cheryl know that the new addition to her family would potentially be responsible for saving her life.

In November 2004, Cheryl, who was 29 at the time, went in for her 11-week follow-up visit after the birth of her daughter. She underwent a Pap smear, which she had been doing for years without any problems. In January 2005, she received a call from her obstetrician's office informing her that her test result came back abnormal, and they had found precancerous cells. She went in for another exam. Her doctor told her not to worry, that it was probably nothing and he could just laser the suspicious spot. Then she received another phone call informing her that the doctor didn't like the look of the results and wanted to do a biopsy. Again Cheryl went in, and again her obstetrician told her not to worry, that it wasn't a big deal, and he would remove the problem spot.

The biopsy went well, as the doctor had promised. He got clean margins when he removed the cancer from her cervix. He said she would be fine. However, once again, Cheryl later received a phone call from the obstetrician's office. The pathology had come back on the tumor, and she had an aggressive form of cervical cancer that could potentially reappear and spread throughout her body. She would need a hysterectomy.

Cheryl booked an appointment at the women's clinic to see an oncologist. When she arrived with her husband, she was expecting to meet with a particular doctor, but instead saw a different one. (This would be her experience throughout her five years of follow-up. She would never see the same doctor or nurse twice.) He told her that she really needed a hysterectomy and asked if she needed some time to think about it. She said she did, and he told her he would give her a couple of minutes to discuss it with her husband.

Cheryl was frightened and worried that she wouldn't be around to watch her daughter grow up if she didn't follow the doctor's recommendations. She has since met other women with the same type and stage of cancer who opted not to have hysterectomies, but at the time Cheryl felt rushed and as though she didn't have any options. She decided to have the hysterectomy.

Cheryl had no further treatment, just follow-up visits. In some ways, this was isolating for her. She was never visibly sick, and it was difficult for people around her to understand how serious and life-changing an experience the cancer was for her. Physically she was fine, but she had gone through significant emotional trauma. She started taking part in programs at the cancer center, such as meditation and art therapy, and started seeing a counselor. She connected with other young adults who had experienced cancer and who could relate with the fear and isolation she felt. It was a relief for Cheryl to finally be able to share her story with people who understood what it felt like to go through what she did. Eight years out, Cheryl no longer has to go for regular checkups with an oncologist, but she remains connected to the young adult community that helped her heal from the emotional wounds inflicted by cancer.

Daylan

Daylan was 18 when he was diagnosed with acute B-cell leukemia. He noticed he was slowing down at work. He was enrolled in a culinary course at the time, and part of his education included working as a cook, something for which Daylan had a passion. He began to have trouble moving bins of ice. Things he used to lift easily were suddenly too heavy. He had trouble staying awake in school and went from being a model student to one who was struggling.

About a month after initially feeling sick, Daylan went to have his eyes tested to see if he was a candidate for laser surgery. The clinician couldn't do the exam because Daylan had too many broken blood vessels in his eyes. He was told it could be a sign of diabetes, and because he had a history of diabetes on both his mother's and father's sides, he went to the urgent care clinic at the hospital to see if he could get some answers. They drew some blood and told him to relax; it would take a while to get the results. Daylan fell asleep, and when he woke up his mother and father were there. The doctor came in and started talking about the blood test results, but Daylan wanted him to cut to the chase. The doctor told him he had cancer. Daylan went numb.

Daylan enrolled in a clinical trial. When asked if he would take part, he figured he was already in such a bad place that he might as well do what he could if it might help others. He became very ill, losing 50 pounds in two weeks. His long, rocker hair fell out, leaving him bald. He was also angry—angry at himself because he thought maybe there was something he could have done to keep from getting sick, and angry at the limitations placed on him by the cancer and the treatment. No longer was he the physically dominant young man who jumped right back up after being hit by a cab. He couldn't go out in crowds and couldn't hold down food. He lost his love of cooking and could barely stand to be around food.

From March 2010 until July 2012, Daylan was on one form of chemotherapy or another to get him in remission and keep him there. He was ready for his life as a healthy adult to begin. He looked into a railway conductor course and met with the head instructor in August 2012. The instructor liked Daylan but wanted him to take more time to recover from his illness before starting the course. It was agreed that he would begin in May 2013.

Sometime in December 2012, Daylan began to feel unwell. His ribs felt like they were collapsing, his back felt out of alignment, and he had trouble breathing. After his scheduled blood tests in January 2013, he received a call to go to the hospital because his blood tests showed abnormal results. His leukemia had come back.

Daylan began chemotherapy again. There is talk of a possible bone marrow transplant. He is back in survival mode, trying to put the fear and anger aside to do what needs to be done. He knows this road is tough, but he is letting the flame of hope light his way.

Note: Daylan passed away in August 2013, shortly before this book went to the publisher.

Gayle

The first thing Gayle said to her daughter, Jennifer, age 29, when she called to tell her mother that she had been diagnosed with leukemia was, "That's OK; we'll fix it." Gayle doesn't know if it was the nurse in her or the mom in her talking—all she knew was that she needed to educate herself about the disease and learn how to support her adult daughter through this health crisis.

Gayle went straight to the hospital to be with Jennifer and her husband as they met with the oncologist. Gayle took notes, her nurse's instinct kicking in, knowing that they would need those notes to remember all the information the doctor was giving them. She turned to her colleagues and the Internet to learn more and read through all the pamphlets and brochures Jennifer was given.

Part of her role as caregiver meant knowing when to and when not to jump in. Gayle switched into nurse mode when Jennifer developed a blood clot in her arm from her intravenous catheter, and again when she had received too much of a medication that led to Jennifer losing consciousness. But much of her responsibilities as a caregiver fell on the mothering side. Gayle brought food to Jennifer and made sure she never ate a meal alone. Together they would watch television and talk about Jennifer's grandmother, who was unable to visit Jennifer in the hospital. While Gayle often found herself advocating for her daughter's care, most often her caregiving role meant simply being a mother who was present for her daughter.

Gayle coped with the trauma of Jennifer's illness by throwing herself into work. Work was normalizing and kept her grounded. She also worked right next to the hospital, so she was able to be there for Jennifer at a moment's notice. This was particularly helpful when Jennifer developed what doctors thought to be a life-threatening skin condition (but was in fact radiation burns). Gayle's place of employment was understanding and let her take the afternoon and next day off to be with her daughter. Jennifer, whose husband was ill at the time and couldn't visit her in the hospital, wrote in her journal that if her mother hadn't been there that weekend, she would have died. Gayle fought for her daughter and brought her strength.

It has been exciting for Gayle to watch Jennifer get well again, but also frustrating and challenging. The recovery process is taking longer than they thought it would. She is closer to Jennifer now than before the diagnosis, although as Jennifer gets stronger, she needs her mom less. Instead of calling her three or four times a day, she calls her three or four times a week. But when Jennifer is going through a rough patch, Gayle is still the one she turns to.

Graham

Graham was 25 years old when he was diagnosed with acute lymphoblastic leukemia. The symptoms came on quickly: pain in his leg and hip that came and went, then pain in his shoulders that wouldn't go away. One morning, Graham fainted after he got out of the bath. His wife ran to call for help and Graham regained consciousness, only to faint again as he made his way to the bedroom. He was taken to the hospital where the doctors ran blood tests. Within a couple of hours, they were pretty sure they were dealing with cancer.

The diagnosis came as a shock for Graham, an active, healthy man who had recently gotten married. He began treatment soon after being hospitalized. The first two chemotherapy sessions helped a little, but not much. For the third and fourth treatments, doctors increased the dose and concentration of the chemotherapy, knocking the disease into remission. Graham had a month off after his fourth treatment before reentering the hospital for a stem cell transplant. He entered the hospital in June of 2010. It would be December before he was able to go home for good.

The stem cell transplant proved to be the most difficult part of Graham's treatment. With the support of his wife and family, who visited him and brought him food, and a strong faith in God, Graham pulled through, even though he felt at times that death would be better than the pain he was going through. A book he read while in the hospital about another young man in a nearly identical situation gave Graham strength. Knowing that someone had made it through the same things he was going through encouraged him when he needed it most.

Things happened so quickly that Graham and his wife didn't really have a chance to think about sperm banking. Although the doctors mentioned it, Graham and his wife were too caught up in the whirlwind of a new cancer diagnosis to consider fertility options. Three years later, Graham is on an immunosuppressant, which prevents him and his wife from trying to conceive. Having children was something they always planned on doing, and they hope still to have a family. If they can't have biological children, they know there are other options to explore.

Graham is now 28 years old with no evidence of disease. He returned to work in May 2012, nearly two years after being diagnosed. Though it takes him longer to perform his duties than it did before his diagnosis, he is happy to be back.

Jennifer

It started with four purple toes. Jennifer, age 29, noticed that in the winter months, four of her toes would turn a deep purple. She was curious about what was happening with her feet and went to a rheumatoid arthritis specialist to have them looked at. The specialist did some blood work, and what started out as a quick, easy checkup ended with Jennifer being referred to a blood specialist at the cancer center. There she was told that she didn't have cancer, but that there was something off in her blood counts and she should continue to be monitored.

Two years later in July 2011, Jennifer developed about 20 bruises all over her body for no explainable reason. She figured something might be wrong but waited until her regularly scheduled appointment in September to see a doctor. She went in for her regular blood testing on a Thursday, and the results were alarming enough that the following Tuesday she went in for the first of five bone marrow biopsies. Less than 24 hours later, Jennifer received a phone call and was told she had an extremely aggressive form of acute myeloid leukemia and needed to be admitted to the hospital that night.

Jennifer called her family and tried to reach her husband, who was out of town. He finally returned her call after three hours, and a distraught Jennifer repeated to her husband what she was told over the phone by her doctor. She didn't know then what any of it meant, though she would soon become all too familiar with the language of cancer. Her husband rushed home to be with her. When he got there, they held each other for a bit, and then Jennifer's husband packed her bag and took her to the hospital.

It was hard for Jennifer, a sociable and outgoing person, to have her life confined to a room and a hallway. Christmas and New Year's passed by, birthdays were celebrated, and babies were born. All these things happening in the lives of her friends and family reminded Jennifer that while her life was essentially on pause, it wasn't that way for the people around her. Jennifer's physical isolation mirrored her emotional isolation.

Jennifer kept journals, four in total, during her time in the hospital. Revisiting them a couple of years after her original diagnosis, she expected everything in the diaries to be depressing. What she found, though, through all the chemotherapy and bone marrow transplants, was an incredible amount of hopefulness. She saw a strength she didn't know she had, a strength that drove her through those days and nights in the hospital. While Jennifer was aware of the incredible amount of strength and support she received from her mother and husband, it took looking back to see that she also provided support to herself.

Jennifer is in remission, but cancer still overwhelms her mind. She will be on immunosuppressants for several years to keep her body from rejecting the bone marrow transplant she received from an unrelated donor. She has side effects from the treatment, including drug-induced diabetes and possible infertility. Cancer is not an experience that ends with treatment. The longest and hardest part comes after. But as Jennifer sees it, her future is big. She doesn't have to worry about what's going to happen. The important thing is to remember that she's here.

Jomar

It was the summer of 2012 and Jomar, a 26-year-old civil engineer in training, was working outside doing site inspections. He found himself growing quite fatigued, which he attributed to working outdoors in the sun all day. But his tiredness continued to grow past what he could handle. Then, one day, Jomar developed a severe headache and began to lose sight in his left eye. He went to his physician who went through a long list of things that could be causing the fatigue, headache, and loss of sight. At the bottom of the list was leukemia.

The doctor sent Jomar home that day with instructions to take some iron pills because he was anemic. The next morning, Jomar awoke with an even worse headache that made him so dizzy he could barely be upright. Luckily his doctor was within walking distance. When he saw how much difficulty Jomar was having, he sent him to the hospital for tests.

Jomar spent the entire day having various tests. His boyfriend was there, as was Jomar's sister, who left work to be with him. Word spreads quickly in Winnipeg, and soon even Jomar's employer came by to check on him. By 2 pm, the doctors were pretty sure that what they were seeing in Jomar was acute lymphoblastic leukemia. They explained to him that they needed to do a few more tests to confirm this within the next couple of days, or he could die.

His family was called in to the hospital. Jomar's sister and employer had left by that point, so it was up to Jomar to tell his family that he had leukemia. He felt like he was saying goodbye. That whole day he was rushed around while loaded up on morphine to ease his headache. The doctors performed a lumbar puncture and a bone marrow biopsy and started him on a steroid regimen. Jomar was throwing up, though he couldn't eat. That first day was the most traumatic and exhausting. It was also the start of a one-month stay in the hospital for the first round of intensive treatment that would hopefully knock his leukemia into remission.

Being isolated from people was one of the biggest challenges for Jomar during his hospitalization. A social person, Jomar is involved in his community in a number of ways and is the cofounder and co-chair of the Downtown Community Residents Association, which brings him close to people and invigorates him to take part in his community. But while it isolated Jomar from his community, his illness brought him closer to his family.

When the threat of death is real and close, it can make things that once seemed important matter less. This happened to Jomar. He came from a Catholic background, and at the time that he was diagnosed with leukemia, he had still not come out. But the fact that he was gay mattered less than the leukemia and being open and honest with his family. He is closer with his mother and sister than he has ever been and has a much more open relationship with his brother. Jomar still struggles with his father a bit—his father is still struggling to adjust to Jomar's homosexuality. But ultimately, what matters most to everyone is that Jomar is fine and healthy.

Jomar has been down quite the road, and he knows there's still a long way ahead of him. While he is in remission and has been able to return to work, he still has two years of maintenance therapy to get through. He struggles with losing so much time to illness, but also feels he can't complain. He has free health care, a wonderful partner, and a loving family. His support system is strong, and after talking with other young patients with cancer, he knows that he is lucky and blessed to have that.

Kim

In 2008, at age 31, Kim was diagnosed with stage II breast cancer. She had a left-sided mastectomy and immediate reconstruction, followed by six months of chemotherapy. She had her right breast removed prophylactically and began tamoxifen therapy once chemotherapy was completed. The side effects of the tamoxifen severely affected Kim's quality of life, and after four months, she chose to stop taking it. She doesn't regret her decision, even after being diagnosed with a recurrence in the chest wall in January 2012.

Kim had surgery to remove the mass in her chest wall. Doctors were concerned that the cancer had entered the lymph nodes and that Kim's disease was metastatic, so she was encouraged to undergo treatment with eribulin. Halfway through her treatment, she was reassessed. The tumor in her lymph node was shrinking. After she finished the remaining cycles of chemotherapy, Kim went through another surgery to remove the lymph node, followed by radiation treatment. In February 2013, she began tamoxifen therapy once more.

Having an estrogen-sensitive breast cancer and being on tamoxifen took away Kim's ability to have more children. A mother of two, she would have liked to have more, but recurrence effectively quashed any chance of that happening. But cancer doesn't define her life. Kim refuses to let it. She views this as a conscious choice: to let cancer either define you or inspire you. Kim has chosen to let it inspire her. This is her responsibility as a mother. How she handles her disease and the difficulties it brings teaches her children resiliency and how to cope with the things that are out of our control.

Living with recurrent disease is difficult for many reasons. The hardest part for Kim is the uncertainty and the lack of control. Cancer in some ways dictates her life. Sometimes she feels as though she is just waiting for another recurrence. When she asked a doctor how to deal with fear and uncertainty, he told her to try to live in the moment, to have hope, and to remember that new drugs are coming out all the time. Kim reflects on that advice, but finds it hard sometimes not to worry about the cancer when she is constantly being monitored and watched for another recurrence. She is also reminded daily of the cancer through her scars and physical transformation. Complications with reconstruction led to the removal of her implants. But although it is challenging, Kim tries to live without cancer dictating her life.

Kim is active in advocating for cancer awareness. She works for a nonprofit organization that raises awareness not just of breast cancer, but of all cancers. She is involved with other organizations as a volunteer and shares her story to help other women facing a breast cancer diagnosis.

As of May 2013, Kim is still watching and waiting. She has scans every three months and continues to take the tamoxifen. She has not had a second recurrence and hopes she never will.

Melinda

Melinda was diagnosed in July 2007 at just 25 years old, but it didn't come as a complete surprise. Melinda's mother, two aunts, and grandmother had all been diagnosed with breast cancer, and Melinda had been tested for the *BRCA* mutation when she was 21. She knew she had inherited the mutation and that she needed to be vigilant about her breast health. Her mutation was documented in her medical file, so when she found the lump, her doctor treated it as a serious matter, and things moved quickly.

Melinda was initially insistent that she leave her breasts intact and have only a lumpectomy. But she saw her mother's oncologist, a woman familiar with Melinda's family history and risk factors, who was adamant that the best course of action for Melinda was a mastectomy. Melinda spent some time talking to her mother and researching her options, and eventually came to agree with the oncologist. For the sake of symmetry and to reduce the risk of breast cancer in the unaffected breast, Melinda opted for a bilateral mastectomy and immediate reconstruction.

Reconstruction proved complicated for Melinda. She had problems with her tissue expanders and needed multiple surgeries to fix them. After a number of infections, Melinda ended up with a wound on her right side through which the expander could be seen. She had surgery to remove the right expander, and once she completed chemotherapy, she had the left one removed as well. For three years after her mastectomy, Melinda was flat-chested and wore prostheses.

Melinda connected with other young women on the Internet and was able to talk to others about their experiences with reconstruction. After having such a bad experience with her local surgeons, she wanted to make sure she researched her options before attempting reconstruction again. She met with four surgeons who performed DIEP (deep inferior epigastric perforators) flap reconstruction before deciding on one in New Orleans, who performed the procedure on Melinda in 2010.

Melinda met the man she would marry on a blind date two weeks before her diagnosis. They had only been on two dates when she learned about the cancer, and she called him up and told him she couldn't date because of her situation. He lived two hours away at the time, and insisted on going down to see her. And he kept going, every weekend throughout chemotherapy. He met her family for the first time when she was under anesthesia for her mastectomy.

Because the *BRCA* mutation increases a woman's risk of developing ovarian cancer, Melinda opted to have her ovaries removed in 2008. This put Melinda into instant menopause. Consequently, she has a low sex drive and physical issues like vaginal dryness. Melinda has been proactive about these things, however, talking to her oncologist and therapist about things she can do to make sex more enjoyable. Her mother, too, has offered advice for this situation, and tells Melinda she has to consciously work on her sex life. For Melinda, this sometimes means being sexual when she isn't really in the mood. But her husband is patient and understanding, and Melinda finds that often the desire kicks in once she and her husband have started to become sexual. Ultimately, working on having a good sexual relationship brings Melinda and her husband closer emotionally and helps keep the marriage strong.

Naomi

Naomi's story began more than a year before her diagnosis. In November 2010, she was diagnosed with mononucleosis. It took six months for the virus to run its course, but eventually Naomi began to feel stronger and more like herself. In November 2011, some of the symptoms returned—fatigue and back, neck, and shoulder pain. Then she began to have flare-ups of severe chest pain. The pain came and went, and Naomi visited walk-in clinics where she was prescribed ibuprofen and muscle relaxants. Finally, in January 2012, the chest pain was so severe that Naomi went to the emergency department. That's where, she says, things really began to start.

Initially, Naomi was mistakenly diagnosed as having fibromyalgia. Doctors were looking for a single cause of all her symptoms, but it was discovered that she had more than one thing going on in her body: an autoimmune disorder that still hasn't been diagnosed and the Hodgkin lymphoma that was already growing in her body. In July 2012, after visible lymph nodes appeared, Naomi was sent for a needle aspiration biopsy. The results were inconclusive. In September 2012, she was sent for a full lymph node biopsy. The Hodgkin lymphoma was diagnosed, and on November 5, 2012, almost a year to the day that her symptoms first appeared, Naomi began treatment.

Naomi was fortunate to have a healthcare team who thought about her fertility and family planning options and referred her to a specialist to learn more. Recently out of a relationship, she decided that freezing eggs or dealing with the legal and emotional logistics of asking her ex-boyfriend to donate semen for embryos was not the best decision for her. She brought a family friend rather than a parent to the meeting because she felt a friend would be less biased and more able to help Naomi come to a decision that best suited her own wants and needs.

Throughout her treatment, Naomi was her own advocate. She found comfort in controlling the things she could, like maintaining her own schedule and taking care of her dog herself when she moved back home with her mother, or by refusing a medical procedure (the placement of a central line) that she was loathe to go through, despite the suggestion of her chemotherapy nurses. Naomi also asked for psychiatric care during the 10 months prior to her diagnosis. For Naomi, the time it took to obtain psychiatric support was one of the most disappointing things she experienced in her care, a failure on the part of her medical team and the health system as a whole.

Having literature about medical studies, concrete information and data, at hand helped Naomi make the decisions that were right for her. With the support of her family, friends, and ex-boyfriend, Naomi completed treatment in April 2013. She is now living on her own and expects to return to work soon.

Robyn

Robyn was 33 and breast-feeding her nine-month-old baby in January 2012, so she didn't think too much of the lump in her left breast when she found it. She called her doctor, thinking it was mastitis, and he called a prescription for an antibiotic in to the pharmacy without seeing Robyn. She filled the prescription and did everything she was supposed to for mastitis—she nursed from that side first, applied heat, and massaged the area. The lump didn't change, though, and Robyn left a message for her doctor or nurse to call her. When they returned her call, they weren't concerned and told Robyn to call again if she had any other questions. This left her angry and frustrated. She waited a couple of weeks before doing anything else.

One night in February, Robyn went to sleep lying on her left side, and her shoulder started to hurt. She thought the infection in her breast had spread, so once again she called her doctor, who ordered an ultrasound. It took two weeks to get an appointment, so by the time Robyn finally saw a radiologist, it was March.

Robyn hadn't told anyone, not even her husband, that she was going for an ultrasound. She thought it would be a routine appointment and she would have the infection drained and that would be it. So when the laboratory technician conducting the ultrasound called the radiologist in and the radiologist told Robyn she would have to have a biopsy done right then, she was more than caught off guard. The radiologist took the biopsy and showed it to Robyn. It was solid, he said, which meant it was either cancer or some kind of benign tumor. She had to call a surgeon that day because she would need to have it removed. The radiologist called Robyn the next day and confirmed that the lump was cancer. A week after that, she met with an oncologist, had a port placed in her chest, and started chemotherapy.

Robyn's tumor was 5 × 3 cm and had infiltrated her lymph nodes, so her oncologist ordered neoadjuvant chemotherapy to shrink it before performing surgery. After each chemotherapy session, the tumor shrank by half, and by July, when she saw the oncology surgeon, it was nonpalpable. By August the tumor had shrunk to 2 mm and the cancer in her lymph nodes was fully gone. Robyn had a bilateral, skin-sparing, nipple-sparing mastectomy. Then, in October 2012, she began five-and-a-half weeks of radiation.

It was hard for Robyn's children—she has an 11-year-old, 9-year-old, and 4-year-old in addition to the baby—to watch their mother lose her hair. Robyn grieved having to wean her baby before she was ready but felt good about donating breast milk to a study that examines the milk of breast-feeding mothers diagnosed with cancer. That's not the only study she is part of, either. Both Robyn's mother and grandmother had breast cancer, so Robyn was tested for all known mutations linked to the disease. She tested negative but donated blood to a facility that is looking for new genes that could be implicated in hereditary breast cancer.

Robyn has found many ways to calm herself and cope with her fears. She takes part in music therapy. She reads a lot, spends time with her friends, watches funny shows, and laughs all the time. And she dances.

Sarah

Sarah was 28 when she was diagnosed with metastatic breast cancer in 2010. In addition to the two cancerous tumors in her breast, she had three metastases in her liver and a metastasis to her sacral spine. Six months of paclitaxel, trastuzumab, and zoledronic acid got rid of all but the primary tumors in her breast. Mastectomy is not often performed on women with metastatic breast cancer, but after searching out several other opinions, Sarah finally found a doctor willing to consider the surgery. She had a bilateral mastectomy followed by eight weeks of doxorubicin and cyclophosphamide to kill any stray cells, and radiation to her chest wall and sacral spine to prevent cancer from returning in the bone.

For nine months, Sarah was OK. Then a scan revealed spots near her pancreas. The cancer had returned in her lymph nodes around the pancreas and then started to spread to the lymph nodes near the aorta. Sarah began treatment again, this time with vinorelbine and trastuzumab. The treatment wasn't working, so Sarah turned to clinical trials. After contacting a pharmaceutical company herself, she was connected with an oncologist at Dana-Farber Cancer Institute and began a clinical trial with an experimental drug. Sarah has been on the drug for a year and a half and has been disease free for more than a year.

The hardest part of having cancer for Sarah has been losing her sense of control. She turns to online communities for support and blogs about her experience. Her parents have been strong supporters as well. But not everyone in her life has been there for her. Communication between Sarah and her husband broke down, and the financial and emotional strain of the cancer diagnosis took a toll on their relationship. They are now separated with an 11-year-old son.

Having metastatic disease does not mean life is over. Sarah struggles to live her life and enjoy what she has without dwelling on her disease. She tries to see this part of her life as a new chapter rather than an ending. And with new treatments and therapies comes hope for an extended life.

Serena

In October 2009, Serena was diagnosed with non-Hodgkin lymphoma. She had just turned 23. Her symptoms were nondescript in the beginning, a slight shortness of breath when she was working out, hardly noticeable. But that shortness of breath increased to the point that even climbing the stairs of her two-story walk-up left Serena breathless.

As the summer months progressed, Serena developed a dry, hacking cough. By September, she began developing headaches and sounded as though she had bronchitis. Finally, she went to see her chiropractor, who sent her for an x-ray and saw what he thought was a harmless heart shadow. By the first week of October, veins and bruises started appearing on Serena's chest. She was unable to sleep on her back because pressure in her chest kept her from being able to catch her breath. On October 13, Serena had had enough and went to the emergency department.

In the emergency department, Serena's heart rate was elevated even as she sat. Her blood pressure was through the roof. The triage nurse knew something was seriously wrong and sent her through to see a doctor. Initially, the doctor thought Serena had asthma and had her perform a spirometry test. She was sent for a second x-ray and finally a CT (computed tomography) scan. After the scan, she met with a thoracic surgeon for the first time. A day later she was in surgery to have a biopsy of an 18×15 cm mass in her chest.

The mass was so large it was compressing her chest, causing the shortness of breath. It was also responsible for her headaches. The mass was cutting off the blood supply to Serena's brain, causing a condition called vena cava syndrome. She was admitted to the hospital for 16 days. On the first two days, Serena received high-dose radiation to her chest to reduce the swelling in her neck to allow adequate blood flow to her brain. She had an anaphylactic reaction to her first chemotherapy infusion. When Serena was finally discharged from the hospital, she returned home to her parents' single-story house rather than to the walk-up she shared with her husband of three years. She lived with them for more than a month before returning to her apartment.

From October 2009 to March 2010, Serena had chemotherapy, eight treatments in total. By her fifth treatment, she had to return to work 20 hours a week. She had only just started her job a month before her diagnosis and lacked benefits. The leasing company made it difficult for Serena and her husband to break their lease, which they could not afford on her husband's salary alone. Eventually, they were able to move into the basement of Serena's parents' home. One month after chemotherapy finished, Serena began radiation and had 15 sessions in total.

Serena used many resources to help her through the emotional and physical turmoil of a cancer diagnosis. Through CancerCare Manitoba, she was able to attend a Look Good, Feel Better session, and she participated in yoga and art therapy. She kept photo and written journals chronicling her experiences to help her process the anger she felt. With her husband, Serena began seeing a social worker, which made it easier for her to share with him how overwhelmed and out of control she felt and gave them a space to talk about how the cancer diagnosis affected them as a couple.

Stuart

Stuart was diagnosed with acute lymphoblastic leukemia in 2001 when he was 27 years old. Initially, he saw his doctor for what he thought was a hernia but was in fact an inflamed lymph node. After a couple of inconclusive biopsies, Stuart was sent for an open biopsy and learned that he had cancer. He spent a relatively uneventful month, with the exception of acute pancreatitis that made eating difficult, in the hospital receiving induction chemotherapy. Stuart had a month off before starting consolidation chemotherapy. During that time, he married his girlfriend, whom he had met about a year before his health issues appeared.

Consolidation therapy was slightly more complicated than induction. A CT scan revealed what doctors thought was a fungal infection. Stuart went through an open lung biopsy, two liver biopsies, and a bronchoscopy before the doctors determined he did not have a fungal infection but was likely having some kind of reaction to the chemotherapy itself. Stuart finished his final consolidation treatment on New Year's Eve, six months after his July 1 induction. After that, he spent three years on maintenance therapy.

Stuart returned to work while on his maintenance therapy. In May 2006, his son was born. Then in the late summer of 2008, Stuart began having brief one- or two-second headaches during which his vision would black out. A neurologist was unable to find anything suspicious on Stuart's MRI and referred him to an ophthalmologist, who measured high pressure in his eyes. Stuart was then referred to yet another neurologist. By the time Stuart saw the second neurologist, it was December— several months after his headaches first started.

By the beginning of January, Stuart's headaches were so severe that he couldn't lie down and he began vomiting. Stuart's neurologist told him to go to the emergency department to meet the neurology team. Stuart arrived at the hospital in the late afternoon and by that evening had been diagnosed with a relapse of acute lymphoblastic leukemia in his central nervous system, seven-and-a-half years after his initial diagnosis. His wife was five months pregnant with their second child.

Stuart spent the next few months in and out of the hospital receiving chemotherapy to bring him back to remission. During that time, he was only allowed home on the occasional weekend, and most of his communication with his 2½-year-old son happened over Skype™. While Stuart was in the hospital, his second son was born. In May 2009, one month and a day after his son's birth, Stuart was scheduled for a stem cell transplant from an unrelated donor.

The transplantation wasn't a smooth ride for Stuart. He has dealt with graft-versus-host disease (an autoimmune complication commonly seen after bone marrow or stem cell transplantation) in his mouth and potentially in his lungs (he is still seen by a respirologist), as well as vision loss from the increased eye pressure he suffered from the recurrence. Treatment left him with low testosterone levels, which led to a lack of sexual desire and added strain to his relationship with his wife. Combined with other issues, some illness related and some not, this contributed to Stuart and his wife's separation in November 2010. While Stuart is once again in remission from his cancer, he is still living with the aftershocks.

Susan

Susan's daughter, Elaina, was a 30-year-old restaurant owner in Florida when she was diagnosed with metastatic breast cancer. For five years, Susan and her husband were Elaina's primary caregivers. Susan would spend hours each night researching metastatic breast cancer online, trying to find out everything she could about the disease. She learned that it is an often overlooked and ignored area in cancer research. Still, Susan advocated for her daughter and acted as a liaison to the doctors and nurses treating her daughter. Through her caregiving duties, Susan was exposed to areas in cancer treatment that need improvement. Access to nutritionists and physical therapists would be advantageous to patients, as Susan sees it, and assigning social workers to work with people with cancer and their supporters would go a long way to teaching partners and family members how to manage and take care of loved ones. For Susan, it's not just about taking care of a person who is ill; it is about learning to navigate a complicated and stressful process.

From the beginning, Susan and her husband made an agreement that they wouldn't take out their anger and frustration on each other, no matter how stressful it got. They knew that in order to support their daughter, they needed to support one another. Susan says it was the best decision they made.

Elaina passed away in February 2012.

OTHER BOOKS BY ANNE KATZ FROM HYGEIA MEDIA

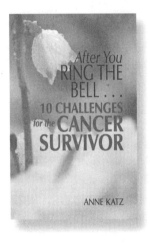

AFTER YOU RING THE BELL . . . 10 CHALLENGES FOR THE CANCER SURVIVOR
A. Katz

For patients with cancer and their healthcare team, the "ringing of the bell" is a significant moment—a point in time that signals the end of active treatment and the beginning of a life after cancer. In her popular book, Anne Katz breaks down 10 challenges often faced by survivors, including health worries, depression, fatigue, nutrition, and the long-term effects of cancer treatment.

ISBN: 978-1-935864-15-8 • Price $19.95

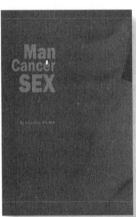
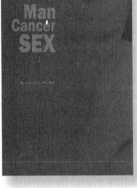

MAN CANCER SEX
A. Katz

Man Cancer Sex explores issues ranging from loss of libido to communication with a partner, discussing all the problems and concerns in between. 2009. 176 pages. Softcover.

ISBN: 978-1-890504-87-8 • Price $19.95

WOMAN CANCER SEX
A. Katz

"A particularly good purchase for consumer health collections."–*Library Journal*

2009. 184 pages. Softcover.

ISBN: 978-1-890504-80-9 • Price $14.95

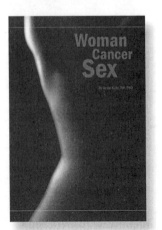

Find these and other Hygeia Media titles at your local or online book reseller, or order directly from the Oncology Nursing Society at www.ons.org/publications.

Hygeia Media e-books are also available for your e-reader, tablet, or smartphone. Visit iTunes, the Amazon Kindle Store, and the Nook Book Store and download today!